Fitness for Seniors

Amazing Body Breakthroughs for Super Health

Publisher's Note

The editors of FC&A have taken careful measures to ensure the accuracy and usefulness of the information in this book. While every attempt has been made to assure accuracy, errors may occur. We advise readers to carefully review and understand the ideas and tips presented and to seek the advice of a qualified professional before attempting to use them. The publisher and editors disclaim all liability (including any injuries, damages or losses) resulting from the use of the information in this book.

The health information in this book is for information only and is not intended to be a medical guide for self-treatment. It does not constitute medical advice and should not be construed as such or used in place of your doctor's medical advice.

No temptation has seized you except what is common to man. And God is faithful; He will not let you be tempted beyond what you can bear. But when you are tempted, he will also provide a way out so that you can stand up under it.

— 1 Corinthians 10:13 (NIV)

FC&A
103 Clover Green
Peachtree City, GA 30269

Produced by the staff of FC&A

Distributed to the trade by National Book Network

Table of contents

Fitness fights aging

Rediscover the fountain of youth

Advances in science and technology have given you the opportunity to live longer than ever before. As a 65-year-old, you can expect to live an average of 17.9 more years, much longer than your grandparents ever dreamed of, according to the National Center for Health Statistics. So what will you do for the next 18 years? Sit and vegetate in your rocking chair or join the active, fun-loving seniors who enjoy life to the fullest? If you want your golden years to burst with vitality, then you need to actively find ways to reverse aging and ill health.

That's where fitness fits in. It's not just about firm muscles, endless energy, or a trim waistline. It's about giving your body the weapons it needs to fight off both diseases and aging. And if you already have health problems, it's about making the most of your situation.

But is being fit really worth all the trouble? After all, nobody ever died from eating junk food or being a couch potato, right? Well, think again. Up to 300,000 people die each year from diseases or health conditions related to a poor diet and sedentary lifestyle, according to a recent report from the U.S. Department of Health and Human Services. On top of that, inactive lifestyles and unhealthy eating habits may cause as many as 14 out of every 100 deaths in the United States.

But here's some good news. Every time you exercise or eat to make your body more fit, you may be one step closer to saving your health – or even your life. It's like dipping into your very own fountain of youth. So why wait? You can turn back the hands of time right now by adopting healthy habits and a "can-do" attitude. It may seem daunting, but think about this – studies show regular exercise can reverse 20 years of aging! And it's never too late to start. Here are some typical "old-age" problems you can slow or prevent with a healthy, active lifestyle:

- Lost flexibility in your joints
- Tooth loss and gum disease
- Some types of mental confusion
- Higher body fat and a slower metabolism
- Digestive problems and constipation
- Increased blood cholesterol
- Bone loss or thinning bones
- Skin wrinkling caused by sun damage

So how do you get these anti-aging benefits? It works a lot like an insurance policy. If you make regular "payments" into your anti-aging account, those benefits can be there when you need them. And every time you eat right, get physical exercise, or reduce stress, you make one of those payments. Like Clark Kent, these anti-aging secrets seem too mild and ordinary to make a difference. But more and more medical research shows that they may have all the power of Superman – just waiting to be unleashed.

Stay young by eating right

A healthy diet is the first step to keeping your youth and vitality. What you choose to eat can make or break the aging process, scientists say. Here's why. Over time, unstable molecules called free radicals can damage many of your healthy cells. In fact, this long-term wear-and-tear on your cells is probably the main contributor to aging. Luckily, your body makes free-radical fighters called antioxidants – power-packed molecules that disarm free radicals and prevent cell damage before it happens.

Unfortunately, as you grow older, your body makes fewer antioxidants. At the same time, irritants like stress and cigarette smoke create even more free radicals in your body. When these bad guys start winning, your body loses, and you fall prey to ill health and disease.

Obviously, the way to stop this free radical overload is to get more antioxidants into your body. Fortunately, healthy foods are full of them. So every time you eat right, you help your body fight free radicals – and maybe aging as well. By choosing nutritious foods and eating them often, you'll help keep your vision, brainpower, strength, and stamina, among other things. And this isn't just a scientific theory cooked up in laboratory test tubes. Georgia's Marcy Walker explains how better eating may have helped someone dear to her.

"My mother lived her entire life on the fast track – never slowing down to eat a proper meal. At age 60, she was diagnosed with diabetes," Marcy says. The doctor's orders were simple. Eat a healthy diet and give up sugar completely. That was 12 years ago.

"She is now 72. She lives alone, works full time, and travels everywhere," Marcy comments. "Fruits and vegetables have taken a very important role in her diet, and she makes time to eat well. At the age of 70, she traveled to Nepal and went on an expedition to climb Mount Everest. I look forward to what she'll do at 80."

Other seniors, who exercise regularly, know that's only half the equation to good health. So they're doing their best to eat right as well. Sixty-six-year-old marathon runner Ann Akers says high blood pressure runs in her family, so she tops off her running with a good diet to help keep her blood pressure under control. "I stick with low fat or no fat," she says. "I watch what I eat." And although 70-year-old Yvette Boucher exercises at the gym for an hour almost every day, she makes sure she eats nutritiously as well. "It keeps my cholesterol down," she says.

All these women have the right idea. Eating well can be a powerful weapon against disease. In fact, it's like a two-for-one deal. The same free radicals that lead to aging can also leave you vulnerable to diseases and health conditions. So each time you eat the antioxidants that may resist aging, you could slash your risk for conditions like stroke and cancer.

Most older Americans have a chronic disease they can fight with good eating habits. Include nutrition in any overall fitness plan to tackle asthma, cancer, heart disease, Alzheimer's, diabetes, osteoarthritis, osteoporosis, or obesity. You may be surprised at what it can do for you.

Exercise to rejuvenate and recharge

You need exercise along with a nutritious diet if you want to reap the full benefits of a fit body. You may groan at the thought, but scientists have proven regular exercise may help reduce – or even reverse – physical losses and aging. In fact, research suggests you can gain back much of the strength, balance, flexibility, and coordination you had when you were much younger. Even if you're over 90 years old!

The first thing exercise does is boost your endurance and give you new energy. If you often feel exhausted, lack of exercise could be a factor. Think about it. When you don't exercise your muscles and your other body parts, they aren't as well-conditioned to handle physical demands. Not surprisingly, that leads you to wear out more quickly. Scientists have nicknamed this problem, "sedentary inertia."

Older adults are making their mark as athletes. Nearly 250,000 people over age 50 compete in state, local, and national Senior Games each year.

But exercise can be the answer – if you stay with it long enough. At first, the extra action will make you more tired because it places new demands on your body. On the other hand, you may sleep more soundly, too. And, over time, your body will grow stronger and get used to this new level of activity. One day you could suddenly realize that you have more energy than you used to – and a lot more stamina. Seventy-three-year-old Mary Zdanowski was surprised and thrilled at the amount of energy she developed after a month of walking the treadmill. "I've gotten to the point where I feel so good afterward that I look forward to it every day," she says.

That extra zip and endurance could help you get more out of every day. It especially comes in handy with the grandchildren, or even, in some cases, your own children. Take 74-year-old "Bob" for example. Late fatherhood has given him new incentive to exercise and stay healthy so he can keep pace with the younger generation. "I have an 8-year-old son, and I've been swimming with him since he was six months old. I want to be able to keep up with him," he explains.

Use fitness as your weapon against aging, and you may also fend off the dangerous health problems associated with growing older. In fact, it may be easier than you think. Consider these examples from scientific and medical studies.

- Walk 30 to 45 minutes three times a week, and you can cut your risk of heart attack in half.

- Slash your odds of type 2 diabetes by 50 percent – with just 40 minutes of moderate exercise each week.

- Exercise may be as effective as medication at increasing good cholesterol levels and reducing the bad. That means healthier arteries, lower blood pressure, and a lower risk of stroke and heart troubles.

- Regular physical activity can help people who already suffer from arthritis, depression, heart disease, high blood pressure, high cholesterol, diabetes, osteoporosis, or excess weight.

Being fit may also give you the fortitude to help fight cancer. Delta pilot Rich Horning is a good example. By matching good eating and exercise habits with his doctor's chemotherapy treatments, Rich defied a cancer death sentence. Surgery was supposed to be part of his treatment program, but his doctor no longer thinks it's necessary. "I have been able to forego a lot of the supplementary procedures and treatments because I've handled the treatment so well," Rich explains. Although there's no guarantee he'll remain cancer-free, both he and his doctors think his fitness efforts helped in this first critical round.

Even if you aren't facing a serious health problem, physical activity may help with everyday pain or stiffness. Just hear what these committed exercisers have to say:

- "I know I have arthritis in the right hip and sometimes it hurts," says Ann. "I trot around a little bit and it doesn't hurt as bad. And the next morning, I don't feel it as much." She believes that even the most limited physical activity can be beneficial to anyone – including first-time exercisers and folks who are physically challenged. "Just a little bit is all they need to do and increase it if they can. It makes all the difference in the world."

- Marcy's painful sciatica forced her to visit her doctor, who prescribed exercise along with an anti-inflammatory. "So I started stretching every morning religiously, and I started doing more exercising," Marcy says. "A week later, I woke up and, for the first time, I did not hurt." Marcy has been pain-free ever since, but she continues to follow the doctor's orders and exercise faithfully.

- Dolores Regan recommends water aerobics as a way to overcome the pain and stiffness of arthritis and back surgery. "I think it helps to keep moving," the 72-year-old Floridian says.

As you can see, a little activity can go a long way towards protecting your body. And you don't have to spend tons of time or money to benefit. You can even have fun. Just pick an exercise or activity that suits you, and give it a whirl. While you're at it, why not spice up your diet with more nutritious foods, too? Then get ready to start counting the ways fitness makes you feel better.

Easy steps to a lifetime of fitness

Are you ready to find out what a fit body can do for you? This guide to health and fitness can help you find out just how easy it is to eat right, stay positive, and become more active. Here are just a few of the pleasant surprises you can expect as you read.

- You'll learn how certain foods can slow and even reverse memory loss, macular degeneration, joint problems, and many more age-related conditions.

- You'll get a nutritionally balanced eating plan that can keep you mentally young and protect you from memory loss, depression, dementia, and other mental disorders. Plus get you in the best shape ever! In just eight weeks, this Complete Nutrition plan could make you feel younger and healthier – all without guesswork or drastic diet changes.

- You'll discover secrets to mental fitness that can help you stay well.

- You'll find valuable advice on preventing and treating disease naturally.

- You'll uncover 20 easy-to-follow steps that can help you lose 20 pounds in 20 weeks and feel as energetic as you did years ago.

- You'll find out how to use nutrition to trim your waistline – along with sensible weight-loss advice and healthy eating tips from doctors and experts.

- You'll get the lowdown on fresh fitness research that may make physical fitness easier than you ever imagined.

- You'll discover all kinds of different ways you can get fit and make fitness fun.

Last but not least, you'll enjoy amazing real-life stories of seniors who have overcome obstacles and stayed happily active. Turn the page and start learning the fitness secrets that can help you live longer, feel younger, and enjoy life to the fullest.

Get fit to feel great

Bill and Lozell Ausman believe it's never too late to get in shape. She is 67, he's 73, and they feel better than they have in years.

It began with a Christmas present. "We gave each other a fitness center membership and vowed we would use it together," says Bill. The decision didn't come lightly. They both have health concerns typical of most seniors.

The couple has found it easy to stick with a routine. "We visit the center five days a week," explains Lozell. "We come early in the morning, Monday through Friday, to avoid the crowds."

"After only a few months, my energy level has increased and I feel more alert, especially when driving," she says. "I've dropped nearly 15 pounds and a pant size." They've both shaken aches and pains that used to slow them down.

Joining together has really helped them stay motivated. "There's someone to encourage you to go on days when you'd rather stay home," says Lozell. "And besides, it's more fun sharing it with someone else. We congratulate each other on our little victories."

Their advice for other seniors thinking of joining a gym:

- Talk to your doctor first.

- Choose a facility that's clean and well-staffed.

- Join with a friend or partner if possible.

- Have a staff trainer coach you in the proper use of the equipment for your fitness level.

Although the cost of a gym or fitness center membership may be a sacrifice, Bill says, "When you realize this is something you can do at a time when your health is probably declining anyway, it's really no sacrifice at all."

Nutrition know-how

Discover complete nutrition in 8 weeks

There's no denying you are what you eat. And no matter how old you are, good nutrition is important. In fact for healthy aging, eating right goes hand in hand with exercise.

Food fuels your body, so proper nutrition is essential to your fitness program. You need nutrients to build muscles and strengthen bones, as well as stay active all day long. What you eat even affects your risk for illnesses like heart disease, cancer, osteoporosis, and even Alzheimer's. Furthermore, proper nutrition can help you manage many symptoms you already have.

Your brain needs good food, too. A nutritionally balanced eating plan can keep you mentally young and protect you from memory loss, depression, dementia, and other mental disorders. It's clear eating right can help you stay independent and active, maintain a higher quality of life, and enjoy a longer one.

The Complete Nutrition eating plan you'll read about in this chapter puts you on that path, without guesswork or drastic diet changes. It's specifically designed to meet the nutritional needs of older adults and lower your risk for many serious illnesses. You'll rev up your fitness level by gradually altering your eating habits one week – and one step – at a time. In just eight weeks, you should feel younger, healthier, and more energetic.

Best of all, the eating plan is super-simple. You start off with a healthy foundation based on plenty of water every day, then build in whole grains, fruits, and vegetables. Add in dairy, legumes, fish, nuts, seeds, and an occasional serving of other meats. Finally, go easy with the sweets and snacks, and you've got a delicious nutrition plan for life.

The Complete Nutrition eating plan

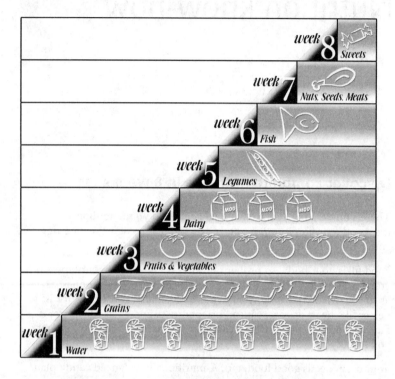

week 8 Sweets
week 7 Nuts. Seeds. Meats
week 6 Fish
week 5 Legumes
week 4 Dairy
week 3 Fruits & Vegetables
week 2 Grains
week 1 Water

Start each week thinking about how that food group fits into your current eating habits. Then slowly make the recommended change – one change per week. You'll either eat more of or cut back on a certain kind of food. By week's end, your new eating habit will feel like second nature, and you'll be one step closer to a healthier, happier you.

This eight-week Complete Nutrition eating plan is designed to keep both your body and your brain fit. It's a recipe for longevity based on well-balanced, age-defying eating habits. The healthier your mind and body are, the likelier you are to live a long, full life – even to 100 and beyond.

Food isn't the whole story, of course. You also need to make healthy lifestyle choices like exercising regularly, getting plenty of sleep, wearing a seat belt, and not smoking. But nutritious eating habits give you an edge. So get ready to maximize your new life and eat for total fitness.

Win better health with water

Explorers searched for it, civilizations fought over it, and now corporations bottle and sell it for billions of dollars a year. With all the excitement over this natural resource, it only makes sense that water forms the foundation of your new eating plan.

In your first week on the Complete Nutrition eating plan, in addition to your regular menu, you'll start drinking more water and other healthy beverages. By the end of the week you should be up and running on eight 8-ounce servings a day. Feeling like a fish? Read on to find out how fluids keep your body in tip-top condition, and what other food and drinks you can substitute for water.

Drink up for fitness' sake

You could survive nearly a month without food but only a few days without water. It's crucial for keeping your body cool during exercise – especially if you're outdoors – and you need it to replace the fluids you lose through sweat.

You can't beat its health benefits, either. Water carries the nutrients you eat to every cell in your body. It cushions joints, regulates body temperature, and lubricates your digestive tract.

It's famous for soothing gout, arthritis, heartburn, and other uncomfortable digestive problems. It can even successfully ward off kidney stones, gallstones, and urinary tract infections.

This divine drink is also a dieter's dream. Water has no fat, sugar, or calories, the units used to measure energy in food.

One serving of water means 8 ounces of:

water	tea
coffee	juice
nonfat milk	
reduced-sodium soup	

But it's no empty-headed beverage, either. It can provide Grade A nutrition, mostly in the form of minerals. Your drinking water might contain fluoride, a mineral known for protecting teeth and bones, as well as magnesium, calcium, or iron. If your water comes to you through copper pipes, you're likely getting more of – you guessed it – copper.

Beware the dangers of dehydration

Unfortunately, many people don't drink enough of this life-giving liquid. Dehydration – a critical loss of body fluids – causes almost 7 percent of the hospitalizations among older adults.

Bottled water or tap?

No water is naturally pure, no matter its source. It all picks up pollutants like bacteria and chemicals. The main differences between bottled and tap water are how each is cleaned and how they taste.

Public drinking water is generally purified with chlorine, which can leave a flavor or odor behind. Bottled water, however, is often filtered, or treated with ultraviolet light or with a form of oxygen. These methods sometimes make bottled water taste "cleaner" than chlorinated tap water.

The federal government regulates both kinds for safety. The Environmental Protection Agency (EPA) tests public drinking water, while the Food and Drug Administration (FDA) sets standards for bottled water.

The bottom line – both are relatively safe, with one word of warning. If you reuse water bottles, wash them out with hot, soapy water to keep bacteria from building up.

Thirst isn't always your best guide, as too many seniors learn the hard way. As you age, your body loses its ability to make you thirsty. On top of that, some medications dull your sense of thirst. People may even deprive themselves of water because they have trouble swallowing, suffer from incontinence, or find it difficult to get up to use the bathroom.

These are very real concerns, but they don't compare to the dangers of dehydration, which can range from irritability to seizures, coma, and even death.

Ignoring the warning signs could be deadly. Learn how to spot these symptoms of dehydration for a clearer indication of trouble ahead.

- dry lips and mouth
- dizziness or headaches
- forgetfulness, confusion
- rapid breathing
- increased heart rate
- dark urine, constipation
- weakness, lack of energy

Toast to your health

You've probably heard the "8 x 8 rule" – drink eight 8-ounce glasses of water every day. But the truth is, not everyone needs that much.

New research suggests you should get eight servings of water-containing drinks or food each day. So if the idea of guzzling eight glasses of water isn't appealing, try substituting an occasional 8 ounces of soup, tea, juice, or nonfat milk.

Making these swaps every once in a while is all right, but don't leave out water entirely. Nothing beats it as the original thirst quencher.

On the other hand, if you're over age 70, exercise vigorously, or have certain medical conditions such as kidney stones, you may actually need eight or more glasses of water every day.

Talk to your doctor about your eating and exercise habits. She can help you decide how much fluid you need and give you other ideas for making water the fountain of your youthful lifestyle.

Get energized with grains

Grains are an energy powerhouse, feeding your body like dry logs on a fire. In fact, most of your daily fuel should come from this food group.

Grains, especially whole-grain foods, keep you fit on the outside by giving you energy to walk or swim, garden or golf. In addition they keep you fit on the inside by toning up your digestive tract. Besides that, nutrients in grains are known to ward off cancer, constipation, mental illness, heart disease, and strokes.

Beginning in week two of your Complete Nutrition eating plan, you'll continue drinking eight glasses of water a day and eating your normal menu, except that, in addition, you'll focus on getting at least six servings of grains a day – preferably whole grains. Servings are often smaller than you think, so they add up fast. For instance, one grain serving equals just half a medium bagel, one slice of bread, a cup of dry cereal, or half a cup of cooked pasta.

Begin making grains a standard part of every meal and snack, and you'll soon meet the challenge of your second week.

Serve up six grains a day

Go beyond bread. Try different grain products like whole-grain muffins, rice, and pitas or more exotic grains such as bulgur, quinoa, and kasha.

Start off right. Make hot or cold whole-grain cereal a regular part of your mornings.

See another side of cereal. Top off tasty casseroles, soups, yogurt, or ice cream with a nutritious serving of cereal. Use it to bread fish before baking or sprinkle it on salad for a satisfying crunch.

Beef up dull dishes. Throw cooked barley, brown rice, or whole-wheat pasta in with other foods like vegetables or soups.

Here's a nutritional snapshot of grains and not-to-be-missed tips on choosing the best ones for all-round fitness.

Power up with the proper carbohydrates

Starch, sugar, and fiber – known collectively as carbohydrates – give grains their get-up-and-go. Without carbs, you wouldn't have the energy to climb out of bed, much less stay fit enough to play with your grandchildren.

Carbs come almost exclusively from plant foods including grains, fruits, and vegetables. Chances are you get many of yours from breads, pasta, cereals, and other grains. But buyer beware – not all carbohydrates are made equal.

Dr. Walter C. Willett, professor of nutrition and medicine at Harvard University and author of *Eat, Drink, and Be Healthy*, warns that the kind of carbs you get from highly processed grains – like white bread and refined flour – may actually do more harm than good.

That's partly because your body digests these refined carbs with lightning speed. Your blood sugar and insulin levels shoot through the roof, and then just as quickly plummet back to earth, leaving you hungry again.

According to Willett, the long-term results of a diet based on refined grains are higher triglycerides, lower HDL (good) cholesterol, and an increased risk for heart disease, diabetes, and weight gain.

Whole-grain foods, on the other hand, undergo much less processing than refined grains do, so they keep more of their original nutrients. The carbs in whole grains also digest more slowly, giving you longer-lasting energy and stabilizing your insulin and blood sugar. Add it up, and whole grains may lower your risk for heart disease, digestive cancers, diabetes, and diverticulosis.

About half of your day's energy, as measured in calories, should come from carbohydrates. Grains are a great source, but choose wisely. Go with whole-wheat pastas, breads, and flour, brown rice, whole or steel-cut oats, and other healthy whole grains whenever possible. You may discover new foods, appreciate new tastes, and perhaps live longer in the process.

Fiber-filled foods: your body's best friend

Grains pack an especially potent punch of fiber, a kind of carbohydrate famous for its health benefits. Experts believe fiber helps prevent diverticulosis, constipation, weight gain, diabetes, and possibly even colon cancer. Fibrous foods also fill you up, so you tend to eat less.

Fiber comes in two forms – soluble and insoluble. Soluble fiber dissolves in water, whereas insoluble doesn't. Each plays a crucial role in long-term health. While some foods contain both kinds of fiber, each provides specific health benefits.

One grain serving means:

1 slice of bread
1 cup dry cereal
1/2 cup cooked cereal, pasta, or rice

You'll find soluble fiber in dried beans and peas, oats, barley, flaxseed, and many fruits and vegetables. This kind of fiber turns soft and sticky in your body, slowing things down in your stomach and small intestine. This gives your body a better opportunity to whisk away harmful cholesterol and absorb carbohydrates more slowly, helping to manage diabetes, for instance.

Your body can't break down insoluble fiber so the bulk of it passes through your digestive system, giving it a healthy workout. This keeps your bowels moving smoothly and tones your digestive muscles, guarding against constipation and diverticulosis. It may protect against colon cancer, too. Look for insoluble fiber in whole-wheat foods, bran, and fruits and vegetables with tough, chewy textures.

Most experts believe older adults don't eat enough fiber-rich foods. The Institute of Medicine recommends men over 50 get at least 30 grams of fiber each day, and women the same age get 21 grams a day.

Get six servings of grains every day to meet this goal. But for the biggest boost, choose high-fiber whole grains instead of refined ones that are lower in fiber.

Folate fends off disease

This basic B vitamin has a big assignment. While fiber shapes you up physically, folate takes on your mental fitness, keeping your wits sharp and protecting you from depression and other forms of "the blues."

Folate also has a hand in building every cell in your body, especially red blood cells, and it may lower your risk for heart disease, stroke, and certain kinds of cancer.

The less refined the flour, the more nutrients it contains. Run yours through a sifter. If most won't pass through, it's coarse and unprocessed enough to lend your body a healthy benefit.

Both women and men over the age of 50 need about 400 micrograms (mcg) of folate daily.

Manufacturers "enrich" many grain products by adding back some of the nutrients lost during processing. Enriched flour, pasta, bread, and cereal have added folate as well as iron and the other B vitamins thiamin, riboflavin, niacin.

A single slice of bread, however, won't give you enough folate for a day. Eat a variety of grain products like fortified cereal, plus plenty of legumes and dark, leafy green vegetables to stay on track.

Antacids and aspirin products can interfere with how your body uses folate. Taking these medications occasionally shouldn't cause a problem, but if you use them often, talk to your doctor about a vitamin supplement. If you smoke or take estrogen, you may need to supplement, too.

Chromium connects with insulin

Balancing your blood sugar can be a high wire act without this trace mineral. Chromium teams up with insulin to turn the sugars you eat into energy for your everyday workouts. While chromium won't cure diabetes, eating too little of this mineral can worsen the disease.

Men over the age of 50 should try to get 30 mcg of chromium a day, while women the same age need at least 20 mcg daily. Whole-grain foods are hands down the best source of chromium.

Just 2 ounces of shredded wheat cereal typically gives you 65 mcg of chromium – well over your daily goal. Nuts, cheese, eggs, and fish are also good sources of this mineral.

Make the most of grains

Work grains gradually into your diet, especially if you eat very few now. This allows your body time to adjust to the extra fiber and nutrients.

Look for foods with these whole grains first in their ingredient list: whole oats, whole wheat, whole rye, whole grain corn, oatmeal, brown rice, cracked wheat or bulgur, pearl barley, or graham flour.

Beware of imposters. "Wheat flour," "enriched flour," and "degerminated corn meal" sound fancy, but they aren't whole grains.

Pick brown rice over white. It's less refined and has triple the fiber of white rice.

Read food labels to find a cereal that contains at least 5 grams of fiber per serving.

Drink plenty of fluids as you eat more fiber to help your body digest it. Try to get your recommended eight servings of water or a good substitute.

Stay strong with selenium

Want to feel young for as long as you live? Then look to selenium. This anti-aging mineral plays a major role in boosting your immune system and making thyroid hormones. It may even protect you against some kinds of cancer.

Men and women over 50 should aim for 55 mcg of selenium each day. Plants, such as grains, absorb this mineral from the soil they are grown in. So six servings of whole grains should provide you with all the selenium you need.

As you progress through the Complete Nutrition eating plan, you'll add other foods strong in selenium to your diet – like vegetables and healthy meats.

Whole grains are a gold mine of many other nutrients, too – protein, zinc, magnesium, and manganese. Just remember to eat a variety of grains for well-rounded fitness fuel.

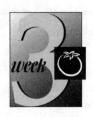

Stop the clock with fruits and vegetables

It's week three of your Complete Nutrition eating plan and you should be used to getting plenty of water and whole grains every day. But you're not through yet. Now you need to add in more fruits and vegetables.

Some foods do more than give you energy – they actually help you stay young. Fruits and vegetables are long-life foods, packed with nutrients to help slow down the aging process and prevent disease.

Vitamins and minerals are keys to healthy aging, and the foods in this group are loaded with both. Even better, most are low in fat, cholesterol-free, and naturally filling.

Unfortunately, the U.S. Department of Agriculture found most people don't eat enough fruits and vegetables to benefit. That's too bad because these delicious, easy-to-find plant foods are a big piece of the long-life puzzle.

Research shows you could drop your blood pressure and lower your risk for heart disease and cancer just by eating plenty of fruits and vegetables.

Getting more home-grown nutrition from these foods is a delicious way to live to 100, and it's unbelievably easy. During the third week of your Complete Nutrition eating plan, begin building in a total of six servings of veggies and fruits every day.

Serve up six fruits and veggies a day

Grow gradually. Add an extra serving at each meal during week three until you reach your total of six a day.

Get creative. Slice up strawberries, peaches, or bananas on hot or cold cereal, or stir them into plain, low-fat yogurt.

Can the meat. Leave meat out of one meal at least twice a week and add more vegetables instead.

Mix and mingle. Toss extra fruits and vegetables into salads, soups, or casseroles.

Make fancy sandwiches. Don't settle for just meat and bread — dress them up with lettuce, tomato, cucumbers, sliced carrots, and green or red pepper.

Dig it as dessert. Try fruit as a sweet end to your meals instead of high-calorie, high-fat desserts.

Nibble all day. Keep a bag of dried fruits or fresh sliced veggies at hand for snacking throughout the day.

Antioxidants: the key to healthy aging

When you cut open an apple, oxygen in the air reacts with it, creating unstable compounds called free radicals. These compounds damage the apple, turning it brown.

The same thing happens in your body. You breathe in oxygen. Your body processes it, creating free radicals at the same time. These travel through your body looking for electrons they can steal from healthy cells in order to become stable. When they succeed, they leave the cell irreversibly damaged. This is called oxidation.

Of course you don't necessarily see the damage as you do with the apple, and it all happens at a much slower pace, but still the harm free radicals cause increases over time. Researchers so far have linked free radical damage to over 200 diseases including cataracts, diabetes, heart disease, and some cancers.

Antioxidants are a family of nutrients that can put the brakes on free radicals. This special group includes vitamins A, C, and E. The minerals selenium, copper, zinc, and manganese, and some nutrients called phytochemicals also act as antioxidants.

These fight oxidation by combining with free radicals to keep them stable – and harmless. But just think how much oxidation is probably going on in your body every minute. In addition, cigarette smoke, pollution, radiation, stress, excessive sun exposure, and other factors can increase your level of free radicals. It's difficult for your natural store of antioxidants to keep up. But you can help. Research proves you can raise the levels of antioxidants in your blood by eating more fruits and vegetables.

The 10 foods with the most antioxidants are:

prunes	spinach
raspberries	raisins
blueberries	plums
strawberries	kale
blackberries	
brussels sprouts	

Arm for battle with vitamin C

In the fight for good health, vitamin C may be your greatest weapon. Don't get enough and you couldn't exercise, and you'd probably stay sick all the time.

Vitamin C is a building block of collagen, the tissue that holds your bones, muscles, and joints together, and it's well-known for strengthening your immune system to help fight colds, heal wounds, and prevent infections. It's a powerful antioxidant, too, so when you eat C-rich foods you're fending off free radical damage.

A woman over 50 needs about 75 milligrams (mg) of vitamin C each day. Men the same age need still more – 90 mg a day.

Citrus fruits like oranges and grapefruit are chock-full of C, but colorful fruits – strawberries, kiwis, tomatoes, and cantaloupe – aren't far behind.

Even vegetables, from broccoli, peppers, and potatoes to leafy greens like romaine lettuce and cabbage, carry loads of C.

In other words, six servings of fruits and vegetables every day should serve you well. Dish out a variety for a delicious dose of vitamin C.

Phytochemicals fight poor health

Plants contain natural chemicals – called phytochemicals or phytonutrients – that protect them from disease, drought, too much sun, and even bugs. Fortunately, these built-in defenders end up helping people, too.

When you eat colorful plant foods, you wind up eating the hundreds of phytochemicals inside them, as well. Many of these special nutrients seem to boost your immune system and guard against deadly illnesses like cancer, heart disease, and stroke. Some even act as antioxidants. Two in particular are becoming famous for their disease-fighting power.

■ Beta carotene is just one of over 600 dyes found in plants. That makes it easy to spot a food rich in this nutrient – look for bright orange, red, or green fruits and vegetables.

As an antioxidant, beta carotene has a knack for preventing heart disease, cancer, memory loss, and rheumatoid arthritis. It even helps save your eyesight as you age.

Carrots, for one, are crammed with beta carotene, as are other orange vegetables like sweet potatoes and delicious fruits such as mangoes, cantaloupe, and apricots. If you prefer greens, dig into the dark leafy variety, especially spinach and collard greens.

■ Lycopene, which gives fruits their red hue, could also give you a long lease on life. Research shows it may protect against prostate, stomach, and esophageal cancer. In addition, it helps preserve your eyesight.

Watermelon, papaya, pink grapefruit, tomato products, and other pink or red fruits are full of this fun phytochemical.

One fruit or vegetable serving means:
3/4 cup juice
1/2 cup berries
1/4 cup dried fruit
1 cup raw leafy veggies
1/2 cup cooked or raw
   vegetables

Scientists don't yet have a general recommendation for the amount of these nutrients you need every day, since different phytochemicals come from different plants. For instance, oranges alone have over 170 different kinds. Cruciferous vegetables such as beets, kale, cabbage, and broccoli are also full of an assortment of antioxidant phytochemicals. Your best bet for all-round health is to make variety part of your daily menu.

Color your world healthy with vitamin A

Also called retinol, this antioxidant vitamin's job is to keep your cornea healthy, guarding your eyesight, particularly your night vision. It also protects your skin, lungs, and bladder from infections and boosts your immune system so you're better able to fight off illnesses.

Women over the age of 50 need about 700 micrograms of A each day, and men the same age about 900 mcg. Only animal foods such as milk, liver, and eggs provide whole vitamin A.

Snacking like a rabbit, though, is another great way to get more A because your body turns some phytochemicals like beta carotene into this vitamin. Look for beta carotene in the bright orange and dark green vegetables and fruits already discussed.

Shape up with potassium

As you hike up that hill, perhaps you can feel your thigh muscles tighten and your heart beat just a little harder. That's all thanks to potassium.

This mineral helps regulate your heart beat, keeps your muscles and nerves working properly, and controls your blood pressure. What that means is you are able to walk, bike, garden, play tennis, and participate in just about any form of exercise you choose.

Fruits and vegetables pack in the potassium, but you can also get it from fish, legumes, and dairy products. That's good news since a fit body needs lots of this mineral. Both men and women over 50 years old should aim for around 3,500 mg of potassium in their diets each day.

A big number like that may sound daunting, but you'd be surprised how fast potassium adds up when you eat a variety of foods. One medium banana, for instance, provides 450 mg. By the end of week three, fit six servings of fruits and vegetables into your daily menu, and you should never come up short.

Keep breaks at bay with vitamin K

Blood that clots and bones that don't break – you may take them for granted. But without vitamin K, chances are you wouldn't have either.

This nutrient makes specific proteins that cause your blood to form clots and works hard alongside vitamin D to strengthen your bones. In fact, a Harvard Medical School study found eating vegetables high in vitamin K could reduce your risk for hip fractures.

People who eat a variety of veggies on a regular basis are usually OK on K. So if you fell off the turnip truck, climb back on. Green leafy vegetables such as spinach and broccoli are the kings of vitamin K, as are lettuce, cauliflower, and cabbage.

All of these outstanding nutrients are just the tip of the fruit and veggie iceberg. This food group delivers nonstop nutrition, including superstars you already know about – carbohydrates, fiber, folate, and selenium – as well as those you'll see later in this chapter, such as vitamin B6 and the minerals magnesium, zinc, and calcium.

Toss together a diet teeming with different vegetables and fruits, and you've got a remarkable recipe for health and fitness.

Dress your plate in these powerful plant foods, and lift your fork to a long, happy life.

Fresh, canned, or frozen?

Food gurus often disdain frozen or canned fruits and vegetables. Their motto: fresh is best.

Fresh, however, is a relative term. Most produce has a short shelf life. After they sit in your refrigerator or in your pantry for about three days, "fresh" foods start to lose their nutrients.

Truth is, frozen and canned veggies and fruits generally have the same nutritional value as their fresh relatives. If you can or flash freeze produce right off the vine, you lock in vitamins and minerals.

The biggest drawbacks to processed foods are the added sodium and sugar. Check the Nutrition Facts label and find foods without these extras.

Experts recommend you buy enough fresh food to last you about three days. Then, switch to canned or frozen until you're able to stock up again on produce.

Make the most of fruits and vegetables

Go for color — dark green, bright yellow, orange, or red are best bets for vitamins A, C, folate, fiber, and certain phytochemicals.

Eat a variety. Different fruits and vegetables contain different nutrients, and you need them all to fortify your body.

Cook vegetables lightly to preserve the important phytochemicals inside them.

Try to eat fruits and veggies whole or sliced instead of always drinking them as juices. Liquids often lack the fiber in the original food.

Don't let mouth or tooth problems stand in the way of good health. Grate, chop, or purée crunchy vegetables if you have a hard time chewing them.

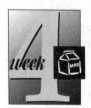

Stay stronger, longer with dairy

By the fourth week of your Complete Nutrition eating plan, you've built a healthy daily menu based on plenty of water, grains, fruits, and vegetables. Now it's time to think about how much dairy you get every day.

You don't have to be young to benefit from this food group. It's the basis of strong bones and youthful activity at any age.

The bad news is one in three white men and women will break a hip by age 90. Blacks and Hispanics have only a slightly smaller risk. While a broken bone is certainly disabling, the worst news is one out of four people die from complications within six months of breaking a hip.

A dairy-filled eating plan and regular exercise could extend not only your independence but also your life. The nutrients in these foods shore up weakening bone, shielding you from crippling diseases like osteoporosis. Write your own prescription for bone health and an active lifestyle by making sure you get three servings of dairy every day beginning in week four of your Complete Nutrition eating plan.

Count on calcium to build your bones

Bones are like a bank – your body uses them to store about 99 percent of its calcium. But your body also withdraws this mineral as it's needed. And it's needed for many functions, sending nerve impulses, contracting muscles, regulating blood pressure, and clotting your blood, to name a few.

The trouble starts when you withdraw more calcium than you deposit. Just like a bank account, you could end up in the red – with fragile bones and osteoporosis.

The solution, of course, is to get enough calcium in your diet to replace what you borrow from your bones every day. That's why it's never too late for more calcium.

Both men and women over the age of 50 should get at least 1,200 mg of it daily. Many experts believe postmenopausal women – not on estrogen – need even more calcium, so they have increased their recommendation for this group to 1,500 mg a day. This is a snap if you follow the three-a-day dairy recommendation.

Dairy foods like milk, yogurt, and cheese are some of the best natural sources of calcium. An 8-ounce container of nonfat plain yogurt starts you off with 450 mg of calcium. Add a cup of low-fat milk for another 300 mg, and an ounce of cheddar or part-skim mozzarella cheese for about 200 more milligrams.

Some cold breakfast cereals are loaded with up to 1,000 mg of calcium per serving, while leafy green vegetables, fortified juices, and fish with small, edible bones such as sardines or salmon can round out your intake of this essential nutrient.

One dairy serving means:
8 ounces milk
2 ounce hard cheese
8 ounces yogurt

Your doctor may also suggest a calcium supplement, but don't rely on that alone to build your bones. Instead, make it part of a healthy, dairy-filled diet.

Fortify your body with phosphorus

This mineral forms the second piece of the strong-bone puzzle. It binds to calcium in your teeth and bones, adding extra might to these hard body parts. It's essential to every cell in your body, not just your bones, for its ability to carry, store, and release the energy you get from food.

Dairy products provide plenty of phosphorus. So you should have no trouble getting 700 mg a day of this mineral, the recommendation for people over 50.

Meat, poultry, eggs, fish, nuts, and legumes also help satisfy your phosphorus requirements — more proof that a diverse diet can help you meet your nutrient needs naturally.

Serve up three dairy a day

Make the switch. Have a glass of milk with a meal in place of soda, sweetened tea, coffee, or alcohol.

Get real. Flavor your coffee and tea with milk instead of instant or non-dairy creamers. And use milk rather than water to make hot cereals, cocoa, and soups.

Jazz it up. Along with your milk, stir plain yogurt into your morning cereal.

Top it off. Sprinkle cheese on salads, soups, casseroles, or hot pastas.

Milk it for more. Add a dash of dry milk powder along with your regular milk in hot foods and recipes.

Rotate in other dairy. Replace milk with low-fat versions of yogurt, buttermilk, cheese, or kefir, a yogurt-based drink. Or occasionally substitute 8 ounces of calcium-fortified juice for 8 ounces of milk.

Snack wisely. Pair up sliced cheese with crackers or fruit for a wholesome dairy-rich treat.

Depend on D for bone defense

You need one more piece to put this strength-saving puzzle together – vitamin D. It is vital for an active lifestyle because it helps your body absorb and use both calcium and phosphorus. According to the American Dietetic Association, your vitamin D intake is a big factor in your muscle strength, fracture risk, and bone health.

Between the ages of 51 and 70, women and men need at least 10 micrograms (mcg) of D every day. After age 70, experts recommend you get even more – 15 mcg a day.

Believe it or not, your skin makes vitamin D naturally from the sun's ultraviolet rays, so being outdoors several times a week is one of the best ways to increase your supply. Unfortunately, your body loses some of its ability to convert D from sunshine as you age. That means it's a good idea to beef up your food sources of this vitamin. Most milk is fortified with it. Cheese is another dependable source of D, as are fatty fish like salmon and sardines, eggs, and fortified breakfast cereals.

Stay away from saturated fat

Fat may be the only downside to dairy foods. Most whole dairy foods are high in fat, particularly saturated fat – the kind best known for packing on pounds, and raising your cholesterol and your risk for heart disease, diabetes, and cancer. But you still need those three very important servings of dairy a day.

Compromise by choosing your dairy carefully. Low-fat and nonfat (or fat-free) milk, cheese, and yogurt contain the same nutrients as their regular versions but with much less saturated fat. They're excellent alternatives for getting your fill of calcium, phosphorus, and vitamin D without sacrificing your overall health.

Compared to whole milk:
Reduced fat milk has 38 percent less fat.
Low-fat milk has 63 percent less fat.
Fat-free milk has 93 percent less fat.

Dairy products deliver other nutrition as well, making them all the more meaningful to a healthy eating plan. So while you're savoring yogurt or guzzling milk, appreciate the fact you're putting protein, potassium, and vitamins like A and B12 in your body, too.

Make the most of dairy

Read the Nutrition Facts label on dairy and other foods, and buy those with the fewest grams of saturated fat.

Realize that not all dairy foods offer the same nutrients. Cottage cheese and frozen yogurt treats have half the calcium of milk. Butter, cream, and cream cheese are mostly fat with very little calcium.

Look for lactose-free dairy products if you have trouble digesting regular dairy. Or buy milk with lactase enzyme added to it.

Shop for soy milk with added calcium if you can't drink milk. Or try yogurt — it digests more easily.

Legumes: love them for a longer life

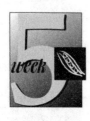

In the story of Jack and the beanstalk, Jack sold his family's last cow for three legendary legumes. This boy knew the value of beans.

You, on the other hand, don't have to sacrifice your family's source of income to share in the wealth of legumes. For pennies a day, you can make them part of your healthy diet.

Legumes are plants that develop their seeds inside pods. Think about how many foods fit that description and you'll understand the variety you have to choose from. Beans, peas, lentils, peanuts, and soybeans all offer flavorful, unbeatable nutrition.

Most legumes are low in saturated fat but high in carbohydrates and healthy fiber as well as top-notch nutrients like protein, magnesium, and the B vitamin biotin. As you see, you just can't beat beans as a high-power fitness food.

Legumes have obvious health benefits like keeping you regular. But there are subtle ones, too. They help control your cholesterol and blood sugar, and cut your risk for heart disease and colon cancer. And they are a waist-watcher's dream, satisfying your hunger longer than most other foods.

During week five of the Complete Nutrition eating plan, add one serving of legumes a day to your healthy menu. With so many varieties of beans and ways to prepare them, that should be easy – and fun.

Pack a powerful punch with protein

Like carbohydrates, protein packs lots of energy, but it's also essential to many body processes like building muscles, bones, tendons, and ligaments – all the parts you put to work exercising. Proper protein can even give a healthy glow to your skin and hair.

There are several kinds of protein, some from plants like legumes, and others found in animal foods like meat and dairy products. Beans alone don't provide all the different proteins, but they give you a strong start. Then you can round out your nutrition by eating foods such as grains, vegetables, fish, dairy, seeds, and nuts – other good sources of protein – throughout the day.

Based on about a 2,000-calorie-a-day diet, men over 50 years old should get 56 grams of protein a day, while women the same age need a little less, about 46 grams.

Serve up one portion of legumes a day

Move the spotlight. Make legumes, not meat, the center of a meal several times a week.

Make a swap. Substitute legumes for a serving of meat or vegetables. Half a cup of cooked beans equals one vegetable serving, while a whole cup equals one meat serving.

Turn green. Add cooked beans, peas, or lentils to salads for fresh flavor and extra texture.

Speed it up. Serve canned, frozen, or fresh beans rather than the dried ones when you're short on time.

Muscle up with magnesium

This mineral serves on the front lines of fitness, helping your muscles contract and relax and steadying your heart beat. It also prevents charley horses, those painful muscle cramps that can put a quick end to physical activity.

Experts recommend women over 50 get 320 mg of this mineral each day and men get 420 mg. You'll fill your magnesium bill easily by following the Complete Nutrition eating plan since most beans are sensational sources.

One cup of boiled soybeans yields almost 150 mg. A cup of cooked navy beans provides another 100 mg. Other plant foods such as grains, spinach, and nuts also contribute this magnificent mineral.

When you wash and peel foods, however, you lose much of their natural magnesium. So, when you can, choose mostly whole, unprocessed foods.

Some laxatives and antacids contain added magnesium. Taking too many regularly can overload your system. Read labels and use even over-the-counter medications only as directed.

Biotin buys you more energy

This B vitamin helps your body transform the protein, carbohydrates, and fats you eat into energy for your daily routine, whether working in the garden or chasing grandchildren. It also helps your body use other B vitamins.

Your body doesn't need much biotin to run smoothly. Women and men 50 years or older require just 30 micrograms (mcg) a day from foods like legumes, cereal, or cauliflower. Peanuts are particularly rich in biotin – just 3 ounces of peanut butter fills the bill for this B vitamin.

One serving of legumes means:

1/2 cup tofu
1/2 cup beans
2 tablespoons peanut
   butter

These are just a few of the big-name nutrients legumes provide. Foods in this family also contain potassium, phosphorus, folate, and thiamin. Then count the minerals such as calcium, iron, zinc, and boron and you've got a nutritional powerhouse on your plate. Make a point to eat a serving of legumes every day during week five.

Make the most of legumes

Cut back on gas from dry beans by pouring out the water you soak them in and cooking them in fresh water. The beans, not the water, hold most of the nutrients.

Soak raw beans at least five hours and boil them for a minimum of 10 minutes. Certain kinds of legumes — such as red kidney beans — are poisonous raw.

Wait to add salt or acidic foods like tomatoes and vinegar to beans at the last minute. They keep beans from softening and can slow down cooking time.

Eat tomatoes, lettuce, citrus fruits, or other foods high in vitamin C with legumes. The C helps your body absorb the iron from legumes.

Add one-fourth teaspoon of cooking oil to a pot of beans to keep them from foaming over as they cook.

Go fishing for heart health

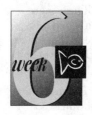

It's not just a leisurely pastime or even a card game. Fishing is now first aid for your heart. Whether you hook them at the lake or at the supermarket, eating fish at least twice a week could sink your risk for heart disease and stroke. And thanks to healthy fats that prevent blood clots and improve your circulation, you could slash your stroke risk in half. In fact, the American Heart Association prescribes fish as a first line of treatment for warding off high blood pressure and heart attacks.

If that's not enough, you'll also do your joints a favor – studies show fishy diets may help tame arthritis. There's evidence, too, that fish could combat diabetes, cataracts, Alzheimer's disease, depression, and a host of other age-related illnesses.

Baked or broiled, fish is a nutritional winner. It's low in artery-clogging saturated fats, cholesterol, and calories, and loaded with amazing unsaturated fats, vitamins, and minerals. So start week six of your Complete Nutrition eating plan by serving up fish at least twice a week. You'll help safeguard your heart and ensure a long life.

Serve up more fish a week

Stick to it. Grill or roast fish kebabs using firm, fatty fish like salmon or tuna.

Wine and dine. Dress poached fish with fresh herbs and wine or reduced-sodium bouillon.

Go gourmet. Bake fish on a bed of thinly sliced vegetables and olive oil. Top each serving with fresh basil and mushrooms.

Make it easy. Add cooked fish to a leafy green salad for a light, nutritious meal.

Polyunsaturated fats perk up your heart

Some types of fat such as trans fats – a harmful kind you'll hear more about in week eight of the Complete Nutrition eating plan – and saturated fat can be hard on your heart and raise your cholesterol. But others known as unsaturated fats actually seem to control your cholesterol and keep your heart young and strong.

Omega-3 fatty acids are a kind of polyunsaturated fat (PUFA) in fish that give your arteries a much-needed break. Experts with the American Heart Association believe the omega-3 in fish can have a huge impact on your heart. Eaten regularly, these super fats:

■ rein in high blood pressure.

■ reduce triglyceride levels.

■ lower your chances for dangerous blood clots.

■ slow down plaque build-up in your arteries.

■ decrease your risk of arrhythmia – irregular heartbeat – and of sudden heart-related death.

But the fats in fish don't stop there. Some experts believe a fish-filled diet could keep your mind sharp as you age.

The protective effects of fishy omega-3 fatty acids kick in quickly. Even if you haven't eaten fish all your life, you could start now and still reap the benefits just by serving up fatty fish twice a week. People who already have heart disease should talk to their doctor about healthy diet changes – like adding more fish – to help get their illness under control.

As you build your heart-healthy menu, remember that fried fish from restaurants, fast food establishments, and your grocer's freezer don't count. In fact, skip these altogether. Fish prepared this way contains little omega-3 but lots of trans fats.

Fish may be the richest source of omega-3 fatty acids, but it's not the only one. Go ahead and up your intake by broiling or baking your fish with omega-3-rich canola or soybean oil, and adding English walnuts or ground flaxseed to your meals.

Iron out weakness and fatigue

It's often associated with strength, and no wonder. Iron is your body's packhorse, carrying life-giving oxygen with your blood to your muscles and other body parts.

If you're low on this mineral, you'll notice. You'll feel too tired to climb out of bed and too weak to face the day. An iron deficiency is easy to fix since, once you're over 50, you only need about 8 mg a day.

Fish, meat, and poultry supply loads of iron for busy lifestyles, and your body absorbs this form easily. Legumes and some vegetables, however, provide a different form – the type your body has more difficulty absorbing.

One fish serving means a cooked filet about the size of a deck of cards. Hint: Fish cooks down, so start with a 4-ounce raw filet to end up with 3 ounces of cooked fish.

Look to legumes and enriched grains to give you iron on the days you don't eat fish. Meats generally are rich sources, too, but later in this chapter you'll read some important information about how to make meat a healthy part of your eating plan.

Be tough with B6

This nutrient knows how to work. It has a hand in building red blood cells, proteins, and even brain chemicals. It regulates your blood sugar and fortifies your immune system. In short, vitamin B6 helps you stay hardy.

Lucky for you it's plentiful in protein-rich foods like fish. That makes it easy to get your quota – 1.5 mg a day for women over 50, and 1.7 mg for men over 50. Three ounces of fresh yellowfin tuna gives you about half this recommended amount.

On your off-fish days, be sure to include a variety of B6-rich foods like bananas, prunes, potatoes, and spinach, or an occasional serving of lean meat such as turkey or chicken breast.

Vitamin B12 reels in better health

Now that you're supplying your body with all those important omega-3 fatty acids, you need vitamin B12 to put them to good use. This member of the B family also works closely with its cousin, folate, to make red blood cells. What's more, it protects your nerves and is a vital part of many natural body chemicals.

If you're over 50 your B12 bill totals 2.4 micrograms every day. That may not sound like much, but your body has a harder time absorbing it from food as you age. As a result, B12 deficiencies are all too common among older adults. That's why experts recommend you pay close attention to meeting your needs for this nutrient.

Animal foods, particularly fish, shellfish, and red meat are bursting with B12. Clams, crab, salmon, sardines, trout, and tuna, in particular, are top-shelf sources. Fortified cereals add their own share of this vitamin to the mix.

Scientists at Tufts University warn that B12 is one of the few nutrients you may need to supplement as you get older. Just talk to your doctor before taking any kind of supplement.

Make zinc your link to wellness

This antioxidant mineral has almost too many jobs to name. It fights free radicals, heals wounds, prevents infections, protects your eyes from macular degeneration, sharpens your sense of taste, and helps your body turn carbohydrates, protein, and fat into energy. Too little zinc in your diet could contribute to poor night vision, lack of appetite, and an impaired sense of taste.

Fish – worth the risk?

Fish aren't the only ones that suffer from polluted lakes, streams, and oceans. When you serve up fish, you also risk eating the toxins they've absorbed.

Fish are the main food sources of the toxins mercury and PCBs (polychlorinated biphenyls). The older and larger the fish, the more toxins it may have accumulated.

Just how great is the danger? The American Heart Association says the health benefits of eating fish twice a week far outweigh the risks for older men and post-menopausal women.

According to the Food and Drug Administration, most people are safe eating up to 14 ounces a week of low-mercury fish such as fresh tuna, red snapper, orange roughy, marlin, and others.

Eat a variety of fish, but avoid long-lived ones like shark, swordfish, king mackerel, and tilefish. Then trim the skin and fat before cooking to reduce your chances of encountering toxins.

Whew! All that work from a tiny amount of zinc. The recommended intake is just 8 mg a day for women over 50, and 11 mg for men over 50.

Seafood is a treasure trove of zinc. Tuna and sardines supply it in small amounts, but the big contenders are shellfish, like oysters, clams, lobster, shrimp, and crab.

If these foods are a little too rich for your taste, try lean poultry and low-fat dairy products like yogurt and milk.

Many fortified breakfast cereals also pack a zinc punch, so check their Nutrition Facts labels.

In addition to the nutrients you've just read about, fish is also a storehouse of protein, key trace minerals, including selenium, copper, fluoride, and iodine, not to mention major minerals like calcium, potassium, phosphorus, and magnesium.

The list goes on, but you get the point. Let fish grace your plate two or more times a week and you'll benefit from its quality nutrition and protective power – important tools you'll need on the road to total fitness.

Make the most of fish

Reel in Atlantic salmon, herring, mackerel, sardines, or rainbow trout for the most omega-3 fatty acids. Pacific oysters are a terrific source, as well.

Serve fish with a side of beans to up your iron. The iron in animal foods helps your body absorb the iron from plant foods like legumes.

Eat a variety of fish to maximize their nutrients and minimize the danger of pollutants they may carry.

Remove the skin from fish before cooking it. This won't affect the omega-3 content, but it will lower the overall fat content.

Buy firm, darker species of fish. They often have more omega-3 fats than fish with white flesh.

Shop for fresh finfish — tuna, trout, cod, snapper, flounder, etc. — that's firm to the touch, has shiny, metallic skin, and no signs of browning or slime. Buy it wrapped in a leak-proof package.

Cook fish with moist heat to make the protein in it easier to digest.

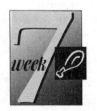

Go lean on nuts, seeds, and meats

For the past six weeks, you've worked on adding wholesome foods to your daily menu. Now it's time to actively limit certain foods that don't bring the same well-rounded nutrition to the table.

Think of the foods in this group as weekly treats – they all make good nutritional additions when eaten occasionally. Overdoing them, however, could be worse than avoiding them altogether.

Nuts and seeds deliver lots of good-for-you nutrients. A few servings each week could promote heart and joint health. Too many on a regular basis, though, could contribute to weight gain.

Meat also carries both benefits and dangers. This food group includes red meat, poultry, and eggs, mainstays of many Western diets. They are full of saturated fat and so contribute to heart-related health problems. Choose carefully and trim back servings, and you can reduce this risk.

One serving of nuts and seeds means:
1/3 cup nuts
1/4 cup seeds
2 tablespoons nut butter

Creating a healthy balance of these foods is your big challenge for week seven, a project you'll take on in two parts. First, learn your game plan for seeds and nuts. Then get the lowdown on meat. Take these foods in hand as you close in on the end of the Complete Nutrition eating plan, and you'll be one step closer to staying fit for life.

■ Gather the power of nuts and seeds

These tiny but mighty foods can actually protect your health. Studies show if you're a postmenopausal woman, eating nuts frequently may lower your risk of heart disease. And both men and women can cut their risk of dying from a heart attack. The nutrients in seeds, on the other hand, can help treat ailments from cataracts and high cholesterol to osteoarthritis.

Both seeds and nuts are cholesterol-free and jam-packed with the antioxidant vitamin E and heart-healthy unsaturated fats.

Remember, though, nuts store lots of energy, meaning they're crammed with calories. That's one reason why a handful here and there could help you stay active, but filling up too often could lead to weight gain.

They are a healthy snack or salad topper, but you don't necessarily need to eat them every day. Just snack on a serving several times during the week to round out your eating plan.

Nuts and seeds are so small they're easy to forget. In fact, your biggest challenge during week seven may simply be remembering to eat them at all.

Serve up some nuts and seeds

See the seedy side. Sprinkle nuts or sunflower seed kernels on salads for a little extra nutrition and flavor.

Live in the raw. Dress greens with raw flaxseed oil instead of salad dressings, or drizzle it on cooked vegetables in place of butter.

Get nutty. Toss a few nuts into baked goods or morning meals like pancakes, oatmeal, or cereal.

Be adventurous. Try cooking with unusual oils such as walnut or sunflower oil.

Mend your heart with monounsaturated fat

Seeds and nuts are chock-full of a kind of unsaturated fat called monounsaturated fat (MUFA). Like the polyunsaturated fat in fish, MUFA helps put a lid on out-of-control cholesterol and shut out serious illnesses such as heart disease.

Studies show it doesn't stop there. MUFAs may boost your memory and help prevent arthritis, high blood pressure, diabetes, and some cancers – no small feat. For extra servings of monounsaturated fat, eat avocados, olives, peanuts, and olive and canola oils.

Experts aren't sure exactly how much of this healthy fat you need each day. Instead, they suggest you replace foods high in saturated fat with those rich in MUFAs. You'll find tips to help you make the switch from saturated to unsaturated fats in the next chapter, *Proven plans from diet pros.*

Stay disease-free with vitamin E

It's added to processed foods to give them a longer shelf life, and vitamin E may do the same for your body. Its anti-aging power comes from a variety of abilities.

As an antioxidant, it prevents LDL (bad) cholesterol from oxidizing and plaque from building up in your blood vessels – good news for your heart health, since that means a lower risk of heart disease and stroke. As it protects your cells from free radical damage, vitamin E may also protect you from chronic diseases and certain kinds of cancer.

It's also linked to mental health and may help your mind stay young as you age. Along with other antioxidants, researchers are hopeful that vitamin E could help prevent Alzheimer's disease.

The most common and powerful form of vitamin E is called alpha-tocopherol. If you're over the age of 50, you should look for ways to get 15 milligrams of it each day.

Nuts such as almonds and hazelnuts, seeds like sunflower seeds, and the oils made from these give you an "E" edge. In general, most strong sources of unsaturated fats carry a healthy dose of this vitamin. Add more E by cooking often with safflower, canola, or corn oils instead of butter or margarine.

Just munching a few servings a week of seeds and nuts scores you other winning nutrients such as magnesium, potassium, manganese, chromium and boron plus vitamins B6, niacin, folate, and thiamin to name a few.

Don't forget to make these foods and their oils part of your regular eating habits, and they'll reward you with a longer, healthier life.

Make the most of nuts and seeds

Grind flaxseeds before including them in recipes, and then use them immediately.

Don't fry with flaxseed oil. It breaks down in high heat and could become harmful.

Many kinds of nuts and seeds contain added salt. Check labels, and choose those lowest in sodium if you're salt sensitive.

Check the expiration dates on nut and seed oils, and follow their directions on storing them. Some have short shelf lives.

■ Get the total story on meat

Steak, sausage, fried chicken, eggs – meats like these can mean bad news for your heart and your cancer risk.

Chosen and prepared carefully, however, meat can be part of a healthy eating plan, just like nuts and seeds. So before you give up on your favorite dish, learn to make it a more wholesome part of your weekly menu.

Red meat, poultry, and eggs are stocked with top-shelf nutrients. They're ripe with protein, loaded with minerals such as phosphorus, selenium, iron, and zinc, and bursting with the vitamins A, B12, thiamin, and niacin.

So what's the beef? Red meat and poultry are also full of saturated fat, the kind that shuts down your arteries and contributes to high cholesterol, heart disease, and weight gain. In some people, high-cholesterol foods like eggs can also raise your blood cholesterol.

A meat serving means:
one egg
2 to 3 ounces cooked lean meat or skinless poultry

Out of this food group, processed meat like bacon, and red meats such as beef, pork, and lamb may pose the biggest health threat – there's evidence linking them with certain kinds of cancer.

In studying the eating habits of over 100,000 people, experts from Harvard Medical School and the American Cancer Society gave their highest "Healthy Eating" score to people who ate red meat less than twice a month.

Your best bet – make fish your main protein source, as you read about in week six, *Go fishing for heart health.* Eat fish twice a week, serve up poultry occasionally for variety, and limit red meat to two servings each month.

When you do include a meat in your menu, go for lean cuts, eliminate as much fat as possible – including the skin on poultry – and bake, broil, or grill.

To make more informed decisions about your meat-eating habits, take a look in *Proven plans from diet pros* for additional fat-busting tips on buying and cooking meat.

Make the most of meat

Substitute a cup of cooked legumes in place of meat twice a week.

Build meals around the plant foods on your plate. Treat meat as just a small part of the larger meal, not the star of it.

Limit meat servings to less than 3 ounces — about the size of a deck of cards.

Gradually cut back meat servings by one-third or even one-half your regular portion at each meal until you reach your serving goal of 2 to 3 ounces.

Choose poultry more often than red meat to satisfy those protein cravings.

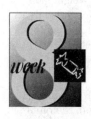

Stay on track with sweets and snacks

You are in the final week of your journey toward better nutrition, and the final change in your diet may surprise you. During week eight you'll learn to examine all your guilty pleasures – like chips, dips, chocolate, or fries – and determine which ones can stay and which have to go. Amazingly, the news is not all bad.

Many sweets and snacks offer little nutrition. Instead they package sugar, fat, and sodium in a tempting recipe for trouble. That's why many eating plans tell you to give up these goodies completely – a difficult task for even the healthiest eater.

But you don't have to forgo your favorite treats on the Complete Nutrition eating plan. Just enjoy them in moderation, choosing versions low in sugar, saturated and trans fats, and sodium. Learn to weed out the worst of them, find healthy substitutes, and enjoy them as occasional rewards for sticking to your fitness goals.

Go natural for your sugar needs

Sugar can give fresh fruits their sweet flavor, or sodas their syrupy taste. The difference is in the company it keeps. When you eat fruit, milk, or even grains, you get a little natural sugar alongside a healthy dose of vitamins and minerals, water, and perhaps fiber.

Commercial sweets, on the other hand, contain concentrated amounts of refined or added sugar, but few nutrients. You'll get quick energy and little else.

Most of the refined sugar you eat probably comes from processed foods such as sodas, cakes, cookies, candies, fruit drinks, and dairy desserts like ice cream. Manufacturers add this extra sugar to tempt your taste buds. Unfortunately, it also contributes to weight gain and tooth decay. Sweet treats can even edge healthy foods out of your diet.

Eating a goody as a reward for hard work won't hurt most people. But indulging your sweet tooth too often can undo the fitness gains you've made over the last seven weeks.

Artificial sweeteners may offer one solution. Saccharin and aspartame, for instance, sweeten foods without adding extra calories. Unfortunately, some research links these sugar substitutes to memory loss, arthritis, and migraines.

How healthy is alcohol?

There's a lot of press about the benefits of drinking – how alcoholic beverages such as red wine may lower your risk for angina, heart disease, and heart attack. Does that mean you should drink?

Alcohol provides lots of energy in the form of calories – so remember that if you're watching your weight – but it contains few nutrients. And it may also contribute to age-related problems like cataracts and memory loss, and can lead to nerve damage in people with diabetes.

The bottom line – weigh your health risks, and discuss them with your doctor, especially if you take prescription drugs.

Should you decide to drink, do so with meals and in moderation. That means no more than 12 ounces of beer or 4 ounces of wine each day for women. Men can generally double that limit.

If you drink more, you cancel out any health benefits and can actually damage your heart muscles and arteries.

Your best bet is to develop a taste for naturally sweet foods – whole grains and fruits like strawberries or blueberries – and eat them in place of snack foods high in added sugar. The next chapter, *Proven plans from diet pros*, offers more tips for spotting added sugars and replacing them with healthier alternatives.

Get the skinny on fats

Junk foods are notoriously high in two types of heart-harming fat – saturated fats and trans fatty acids. A snack made with these bad fats has a longer shelf life than those made with unsaturated fats. That translates into more money for the manufacturers. But if you eat foods full of these fats, your own "shelf life" could get significantly shorter.

Although it's mostly found in animal foods like meat and dairy products, saturated fat also shows up in tropical oils often used to make snack foods – palm, palm kernel, and coconut oils. Surprisingly, coconut oil contains even more saturated fat than pure cream and may significantly raise your risk for heart disease.

Trans fats are an elephant of a different color. During processing, manufacturers turn some of a food's unsaturated fat into saturated fat – to extend shelf life or change the taste or texture of that food. Trans fatty acids are one of the by-products. This unusual kind of super fat raises your cholesterol as well as your risk for heart disease and possibly cancer.

Some treats are top suspects for trans and saturated fats. Think twice before eating these:

- most margarines, shortenings, and peanut butters

- fast food and fried foods including chicken, fish, and french fries

- bakery goods like doughnuts, rolls, biscuits, cakes, and cookies

- chips, corn snacks, and crackers

- salad dressing and mayonnaise

In addition, beware of food with "hydrogenated" or "partially hydrogenated" oil in the ingredients list. These are code words for trans fats. Learn more about spotting and replacing harmful fats with healthy ones in the next chapter, *Proven plans from diet pros*.

Sodium: a little goes a long way

It's a major mineral in salt, and a major enemy to your heart. While some foods naturally contain small amounts of sodium, most of it gets added during cooking or processing to boost flavor.

Salt lends a hand in regulating your body fluids and blood pressure, and helps muscles and nerves work properly. You only need a tiny bit of sodium to get these jobs done — about 600 milligrams or less than one-fourth teaspoon of salt. Most people, however, get over 3,000 mg of sodium daily.

If you eat too much salt, your kidneys, which regulate the mineral and water balance in your body, must work harder to flush out the extra sodium. Unfortunately, a lot of other important minerals, like calcium, get flushed out as well. The more salt you eat, the more calcium you lose. The more calcium you lose, the greater your bone loss and your risk for osteoporosis.

Limiting your sodium to less than 2,400 mg a day — about one teaspoon of salt — could not only slow down this calcium loss but also put a lid on high blood pressure. People who are salt-sensitive and already have high blood pressure could especially benefit from eating less salt.

Naturally, the best way to cut back sodium is to limit salt and salty foods. If you're a snacker, you may find that especially difficult. Read the Nutrition Facts label on foods to discover the sodium content. Then check out the next chapter, *Proven plans from diet pros,* for salt-savvy ways to lower sodium without losing flavor.

Make the most of sweets and snacks

Skip junk food and sugary sodas, and snack on vegetables, whole grains, fruits, and low-fat dairy products instead.

Serve snacks and treats well before mealtime so as not to ruin your appetite for healthier foods.

Go easy on portions. Remember, these are snacks, not full-fledged meals.

Snacking can be a healthy habit. It helps maintain steady blood sugar and energy levels to keep you active throughout your day. It's all in what and how much you eat.

Don't lose hope if you slip every once in a while and go overboard with your favorite snack or sweet. Just remember the healthy habits you've practiced over the last seven weeks and climb back on your long-life eating plan.

Eating for optimal health is not about going to extremes. It's about getting the nutrients you need and finding a balance in your food lifestyle. You don't have to deprive yourself. You can eat the foods you love and still stay healthy. Just follow the guidelines in your Complete Nutrition eating plan and these four golden rules of good nutrition:

- **Adequacy.** Get enough vitamins, minerals, and energy from the food you eat each day to replace what you lose through daily activities.

- **Moderation.** So what if you still love sweets and can't give up red meat. Learn restraint. Enjoy an occasional treat alongside lots of nutritious foods, but monitor unhealthy fats, sugar, and cholesterol.

- **Balance.** While you may have a few favorite foods and food groups, make sure you eat from all of them. For instance, don't ignore calcium-rich foods in favor of those high in iron. You need a healthy balance of nutrients from many different kinds of foods.

- **Variety.** No single food or food group provides all the nutrients you need to stay healthy. Fill your plate with an ever-changing variety of different foods. You'll serve up perfect portions of crucial nutrients and make mealtimes more enjoyable.

Foods are by far the healthiest, most natural way to get quality nutrition. As you age, however, your body's needs change, and you may require more of certain nutrients than you can get from food. According to experts, seniors, in particular, may need extra vitamins D and B12 as well as calcium.

Do your best to fill your nutritional bill with food. Then discuss dietary supplements with your doctor – they are serious business, just like medications. Too much of certain vitamins or minerals can be toxic or mask other illnesses and deficiencies.

In addition to a well-rounded eating plan, some people may need a multivitamin. Again, talk to your doctor about which one fits your lifestyle.

Defend your health with food safety

Total fitness includes not only diet and exercise, but food safety as well, especially since foodborne diseases like hepatitis A and *E. coli* are growing concerns.

Bacteria that sneak into your food may be the most dangerous additive of all. But you can avoid this unhealthy scenario by following a few simple safety rules.

- Wash your hands under warm, soapy water for 20 seconds before and after handling food. Wash cutting boards, counter tops, and utensils with hot, soapy water right after using them.

- Separate raw meats from other foods when you buy, store, and cook them. And make sure their juices don't drip into other foods.

- Test the temperature of cooked items with a food thermometer. Reheat leftovers to at least 165 degrees.

- Refrigerate perishables within two hours of buying them, or within one hour on days when it's above 90 degrees. Refrigerate leftovers within two hours of cooking them, and eat them within three to four days.

Follow these tips as you prepare healthy meals on your Complete Nutrition eating plan, and you'll be one step closer to your personal fitness goal.

Proven plans from diet pros

3

5 ways to eat better and smarter

What could be the next best thing to a fountain of youth – a proven eating plan that is easy to prepare, tastes great, and is good for you. You'll discover five of them in the following pages, along with tips to make them work for you. They're all proven in scientific studies or backed by the latest medical research, they are good for your heart, and contain the foods you love to eat.

Discuss these diets with your doctor before giving them a trial run. She can help you decide which will work best for you and can monitor your progress along the way. In addition, realize that an eating plan alone won't improve your health. You must make lifestyle changes, too – exercise daily, reduce stress, and quit smoking.

DASH high blood pressure with 6 simple moves

If you want to make big improvements in your blood pressure, without the help of medication, Dietary Approaches to Stop Hypertension (DASH) could be your dream diet.

DASH-Sodium, a new study funded by the National Heart, Lung, and Blood Institute (NHLBI), proves a diet high in wholesome plant foods and low in salt can do just that.

Best of all, the results show this diet could work for almost everyone – men and women, young people and seniors, white and black, overweight and normal weight, physically active and sedentary, and even those who don't yet have clinically high blood pressure.

About 400 people tried several combinations of diets and salt levels to see which worked best. Those who experienced the biggest improvement in their blood pressure were people who followed the DASH eating plan and cut back their sodium to approximately 1,200 milligrams (mg) a day. They saw as much as an 11-point drop in their systolic pressure, and almost a 6-point drop in their diastolic pressure – and all without medication.

The DASH-Sodium diet isn't too different from the Complete Nutrition eating plan you learned about in the *Nutrition know-how* chapter. You'll just eat even more fruits, vegetables, and whole grains, and take special care to limit your salt.

People generally experienced the greatest improvement in the first four weeks. But there's more good news – researchers think sticking to a low-sodium diet could keep reducing your blood pressure long after that.

Even if your pressure only drops a little, experts believe following the DASH-Sodium diet long-term could protect you from the slow rise in blood pressure that often comes with age, thus lowering your risk for heart-related death.

The secret lies in the one-two punch of a diet packed with nutrients like potassium, magnesium, calcium, fiber, and protein, but short on salt, saturated fat, cholesterol, and certain foods including red meat, sugary drinks, and sweets.

Check out these basic tips to start putting the lid on high blood pressure. Then flip back to the *Nutrition know-how* chapter for hints on picking and preparing the healthiest versions of these foods. These serving recommendations apply to a 2,000-calorie-a-day diet.

- **Get moving with grains.** Whole grains provided up to half the fiber, protein, calcium, magnesium, potassium, folate, and zinc that people in the DASH-Sodium study ate. To reach similar goals, eat seven to eight servings of whole grain-products – not refined – every day.

- **Fill up on fresh fruit.** Fruits are an excellent source of potassium, a mineral that may help control your blood pressure. Eating at least four to five servings daily will help you get the large amounts of potassium prescribed by the DASH diet.

- **Munch on more vegetables.** Strive for four to five servings of vegetables each day. They provide about 15 percent of the magnesium, potassium, and calcium you get on the DASH diet, and they're terrific sources of fiber, folate, and vitamins A, C, and E.

- **Develop a taste for dairy.** Make two to three servings a part of your daily plan – just be sure you choose the low-fat kinds.

- **Eat fish, poultry, and other meats sparingly.** Under the DASH plan you should limit these meats to no more than two servings a day. Make a point of choosing fish and poultry more often than red meat, and treat them as one part of your meal, not the main course.

- **Add a few legumes, nuts, and seeds.** They deliver even more of the nutrients important to DASH like protein, potassium, magnesium, and fiber. Serve up four to five servings of legumes a week along with a handful of nuts or seeds for a tasty snack.

People who eat a typical American diet get most of their energy from refined grains, fats, sweets, and oils. On the DASH diet, however, your energy comes from more heart-friendly whole grains, fruits, and low-fat dairy products. This diet also gives you more vitamins, thanks to all those extra fruits and vegetables.

Following these serving guidelines isn't the full story. Remember, you also need to watch your salt and trim saturated fat and cholesterol from your daily food choices.

Later in this chapter you'll find quick tips for cutting back on salt and trimming saturated fat from your diet.

Researchers warn that reducing your sodium to about 1,200 mg a day – the lowest and most effective level in the study – can be tough. But the results may be worth it, especially for people over 45 who benefited the most from lowering their sodium.

Talk to your doctor before making any major changes to your eating habits, however. She may have other suggestions for naturally capping your blood pressure.

You can also order a free copy of *Facts About the DASH Eating Plan.* This pamphlet from the National Heart, Lung, and Blood Institute contains sample menus and details about the original DASH diet study.

Just call their Health Information Center at 301-592-8573 or visit them on the Internet at <www.nhlbi.nih.gov>.

Take 2 steps toward lower cholesterol

Is high cholesterol threatening your heart health? Bring it down one step at a time using one of the Step diets – eating plans developed by the National Institutes of Health.

While your body needs cholesterol to help make vitamin D, hormones, and even digestive juices, a little goes a long way. And most people have far more cholesterol than they need, especially the dangerous kind called low-density lipoprotein (LDL) cholesterol.

Excess cholesterol travels to the walls of your arteries and causes fatty build-up, a condition called atherosclerosis. This significantly raises your risk of angina, stroke, and heart attacks.

That's where Step comes in. Endorsed by both the American Heart Association and the National Cholesterol Education Program (NCEP), the Step program guides you through simple diet changes proven to reduce your LDL cholesterol.

Foods containing saturated fat and animal-based cholesterol can send your blood cholesterol skyrocketing. To rein it in, the Step diets encourage you to cut back on these foods and build a better balance of fibrous, nutrient-rich foods.

The Step eating plan has two levels – Step I, a preventive diet for people who need to lower their cholesterol but don't yet suffer from heart disease; and Step II, for those at high risk for heart disease or who already have it. Generally, Step II is stricter than Step I, but both can help lower your cholesterol.

Check the fat and cholesterol amounts on food nutrition labels to be sure you keep within your range.

Remember, the guidelines depend on how many calories you tend to eat each day. As your calories change, so does the amount of fat you can eat. Some larger or very active people may eat up to 2,400 calories a day, while those who are petite or less active may only need around 1,500 calories.

The following quick comparison of the two diets should give you an idea of your daily goals for fat, cholesterol, and calories under each program.

	Step I	Step II
Saturated fat	no more than 8 to 10 percent of your daily calories	no more than 7 percent of your daily calories
Total fat	less than 30 percent of your daily calories	less than 30 percent of your daily calories
Cholesterol	less than 300 mg each day	less than 200 mg each day
Calories	a controlled amount to keep a healthy weight	a controlled amount to keep a healthy weight

Now here's a breakdown of the saturated and total fat you're allowed under each Step diet based on your daily calories. The fat here is measured in grams. To convert that to calories, just multiply the number of fat grams by nine – since 1 gram of fat has 9 calories.

Saturated fat grams per day

Calories	1,500	1,700	1,900	2,100	2,300
Step I at 9%	15	17	19	21	23
Step II at 6%	10	11	13	14	15

Total fat grams per day

Steps I & II at 30%	50	57	63	70	77

Let's say you lower the amount of saturated fat calories you eat every day by just 1 percent. That lowers your body's LDL cholesterol by 1 percent.

Every 1 percent drop in your cholesterol results in a 2 percent decrease in your risk of heart attack. Research shows the Step II diet could lower your cholesterol between 5 and 20 percent, while Step I may yield more modest results. Not bad for such a small change in diet.

These guidelines on specific food groups will help you stay in "step."

■ **Harvest a healthier heart.** Plant foods form the foundation of the Step diets, proving you can best lower your cholesterol by grazing on plants rather than gorging on meats.

Grains and legumes are full of fiber and naturally lower your cholesterol. Fruits and vegetables deliver their own fiber punch alongside key vitamins, minerals, and antioxidants. Plus, most are amazingly low in sodium, calories, and saturated fat.

■ **Get the deal on dairy.** As an animal food, dairy products can be loaded with saturated fat. Make the switch to low-fat dairy like skim or 1 percent milk, nonfat yogurt, and low-fat cheese and ice cream. You'll get crucial nutrients without the danger of excess fat.

■ **Pick winning fish, poultry, and meat.** Red and processed meats are major sources of saturated fat. Buy the leanest cuts you can, and opt for fish and poultry. Even then, keep your portions small – less than 6 ounces a day. That's equal in size to about two decks of playing cards.

■ **Give eggs a break.** Egg yolks pack a double punch – they are notoriously high in both saturated fat and cholesterol. Although it's the fat, not the cholesterol, that does the most damage.

Step I allows you to eat up to four egg yolks in a week. Step II is stricter, limiting you to two yolks each week. Remember, you probably get more eggs than you think – they're hidden in all kinds of baked goods. So skip the yolks altogether and cook with egg whites or an egg substitute when possible.

■ **Know your oils.** Prepare foods with monounsaturated fatty oils such as olive and canola, or with polyunsaturated oils like safflower, corn, and soybean. These seem to help lower your cholesterol if you use them in small amounts. But don't overdo it – they still contribute to your total fat calories.

The National Heart, Lung, and Blood Institute (NHLBI) offers several pamphlets on controlling your cholesterol and improving your heart health. Two in particular, NIH Publication No. 97-3805 and 94-2920, discuss the Step diets.

For more information, call their Information Center at 301-592-8573, visit them on the Internet at <www.nhlbi.nih.gov>, or write them at:

NHLBI Information Center
P.O. Box 30105
Bethesda, MD 20824-0105

Discuss the Step program with your doctor, a registered dietitian, or a nutrition specialist. They can track your results, give you tips, and encourage you to stick with it. Get going, and take the first step toward lowering your cholesterol.

Reverse heart disease with Ornish

Do you want the blood pressure benefits of DASH with the cholesterol results of the Step program? Then you want the diet designed by Dr. Dean Ornish.

He is the author of *Dr. Dean Ornish's Program for Reversing Heart Disease,* a lifestyle program that advocates daily aerobic exercise; daily stress reduction; and a very low-fat, vegetarian diet. Ornish is more extreme than either the DASH or Step diets, but the results could save your life.

In one program Ornish conducted, over 80 percent of the participants managed to reverse their heart disease in less than a year – without drugs or surgery.

In some cases, this program has successfully lowered LDL cholesterol by nearly 40 percent and practically erased angina. Plus, it's been so effective as a treatment for high blood pressure, Ornish had to reduce or discontinue blood pressure medicine in three different studies.

You don't even have to count calories or grams of fat. Ornish believes what you eat is more important than how much. But you do have to choose your foods very carefully to earn the health rewards he promises.

■ **Cut the meat.** To follow the program, you must avoid all meats and most animal products – except for egg whites and a cup of nonfat yogurt or milk every day. Bypassing these foods lowers your saturated fat and cholesterol intake, an important part of the Ornish diet.

■ **Load up on vegetables.** By skipping meat, you create more room on your plate and in your stomach for heart-healthy plant foods. Fruits, vegetables, legumes, and grains bring you lots of fiber, calcium, protein, and other nutrients without the fat and cholesterol of animal products.

- **Say sayonara to sugar.** It won't necessarily contribute to heart disease, but sugar shows up in foods that are also full of saturated fat and cholesterol. Avoid sugary foods and you may miss the others as well.

- **Skip the salt.** You already know it raises your blood pressure, so it only makes sense to cut salt as much as possible under the Ornish plan. Take a peek at the tips for limiting sodium later in this chapter.

- **Lose the fat.** Ornish tells you to give up all oils and fatty foods – even those full of mono- and polyunsaturated fats, not just saturated fats. That eliminates avocados, olives, nuts, seeds, and their oils from your grocery list, too. Leaving out meat and most other animal foods will also aid your fat-lowering crusade.

  The goal here is to keep your total fat under 10 percent of your daily calories. This is a drastic reduction compared to the 30 percent of fat you're allowed under the Step diets.

  Trimming this much can be tough, but keep yourself motivated by remembering how well the Ornish program seems to work. You'll find great hints on limiting saturated and trans fats later on in this chapter.

- **Lower cholesterol.** This program advises you to cut the cholesterol you eat to under 5 milligrams (mg) a day – even less than the amount recommended in the Step II diet.

  Limiting all fats and animal foods, and making meals out of plant foods will help you meet this goal. Read the Nutrition Facts label on food for the cholesterol content.

- **Can the caffeine.** It may add to stress and worsen irregular heart-beats – bad news for people with heart ailments.

- **Watch the alcohol.** Some studies suggest it's good for your heart, but according to Ornish you should limit alcohol to less than 2 ounces a day – about half a glass of wine.

Follow the program closely for at least three weeks before judging its benefits. Ornish claims it takes that long to break old eating habits and establish new ones. Get advice from your doctor before trying this diet, and ask her for more details.

Learn label lingo

Food labels can be confusing — or even misleading. To help you out, the government has established definitions for terms used on food labels. Know what these terms mean so you know what you're getting.

- **Serving size.** The size may be much smaller or much larger than what you consider a single serving. Remember this when reading any "per serving" figures.

- **Fat-free.** Less than 0.5 grams (g) of fat per serving.

- **Sugar-free.** Less than 0.5 g of sugar per serving. The term "low sugar" isn't regulated and may or may not mean what you expect.

- **Low-fat.** No more than 3 grams of fat per serving.

- **Good source of calcium.** At least 100 milligrams (mg) of calcium per serving. A "good source" of a nutrient must have 10 to 19 percent of the recommended daily value. An "excellent source" must have at least 20 percent.

- **Reduced.** At least 25 percent less fat, saturated fat, sodium, cholesterol, sugar, or calories per serving than the regular food.

- **Light or lite.** One-third fewer calories or half the fat of the higher-calorie, higher-fat food. Or half the sodium of a low-calorie, low-fat food.

- **Lean.** Less than 10 g of fat, 4 g of saturated fat, and 95 mg of cholesterol per serving of fish, poultry, or meats.

The Mediterranean secret to a super-long life

People in Mediterranean countries like Greece live longer and suffer fewer diseases than anywhere else on earth. And even though their cholesterol may not be that much lower, fewer die from heart disease or suffer from other chronic illnesses.

Their long, healthy lives have made them famous and given doctors a reason to celebrate. Now you can, too. Experts have devised an amazing Mediterranean food pyramid based on the traditional eating habits of people in this part of the world. Studies show it seems to protect you from heart disease and certain kinds of cancer.

It's also easy to follow. You don't have to make any drastic diet changes – like cutting out all fat or carbohydrates. You can still eat pasta, cheese, even red meat. The key lies in moderation and in eating lots of whole, unprocessed foods.

The traditional Greek diet is full of fibrous fruits and vegetables, unrefined carbohydrates from whole grains and legumes, and heart-healthy monounsaturated fats from olive oil. At the same time, Greeks tend to get less saturated fat from animal foods. The result is an eating plan proven to lower LDL cholesterol and ward off heart disease.

Plants – not animal foods – make up the main part of Mediterranean meals. A plate heavy with fresh fruits, legumes, simple vegetables, and whole-grain pastas and breads sits in the middle of this healthy table. Some experts believe the nutrients in these whole plant foods – fiber, antioxidants, and unrefined carbohydrates – lend the Mediterranean diet its protective effects. Here's how to snag the same benefits.

- **Pick lots of produce.** Put a variety of fruits and vegetables at the top of your grocery list, and eat between seven and 10 servings of them each day. Lay off the heavy cream and butter sauces. Opt instead for steaming or stir-frying vegetables in olive oil.

- **Go for the grains.** Add whole-grain breads, cereals, and other unrefined grains like brown rice, couscous, bulgur, or polenta for a hefty dose of fiber. Avoid refined grains such as white bread, biscuits, and sweet, buttery baked goods.

- **Buy into beans.** Make legumes and tree nuts a regular part of your day. Soybeans, peas, lentils, and other beans are top-notch legumes, while walnuts, almonds, and pecans are excellent nut choices. Just stay away from the salted and honey-roasted varieties.

■ **Land more fish and chicken.** Fish are particularly kind to your heart and may account for the unusually good health people on the Mediterranean diet enjoy. Fatty fish like salmon, trout, and herring supply you with much-needed omega-3 fatty acids, a type of polyunsaturated fat. In addition, work in an occasional serving of skinless, low-fat poultry during the week.

■ **Reduce the red meat.** Plan beef and other red meats as a treat a few times a month. Skip fatty or processed meats like sausage and bacon, and limit your eggs to just a few each week.

■ **Decrease your dairy.** If you lived in the Mediterranean region, you might not have access to cow's milk every day. Greeks tend to eat yogurt and cheese made from goat and sheep milk, which has a stronger flavor – so a little goes a long way.

In fact, while Western diets emphasize dairy products for bone health, Greeks eat dairy more sparingly. This also cuts back on the saturated fat in their diet. You can keep your dairy by choosing low-fat versions such as skim milk and nonfat yogurt whenever possible. But learn to skip high-fat ice cream, cheese, and whole milk.

■ **Load up on olive oil.** To the Greeks, this oil is almost a food group in itself. People from this part of the world often use it in place of other cooking oils, fats, butter, and dressings – and research suggests you should, too. Studies prove the monounsaturated fats in olive oil lower LDL and raise HDL cholesterol, clearing fat deposits out of your arteries and lowering your risk of heart attack.

It's not enough, though, to simply add olive oil to your diet. You need to use it instead of harmful saturated and trans fats like butter, margarine, shortening, lard, and corn oil. Extra virgin olive oil is the best kind. Make the switch, and you could be singing a happy 100th birthday to yourself.

■ **Watch out for other fats.** Saturated and trans fats pose an alarming threat to your health, as you read in the *Nutrition know-how* chapter. Luckily, they make up only a small amount of the energy, or calories, you eat each day on the Mediterranean diet.

Cutting back on fatty meats; replacing butter and other fats with olive oil; and building meals out of whole, unprocessed plant foods goes a long way to putting a lid on saturated and trans fats in your diet.

■ **Snack on fewer sweets.** Sweet snacks and sugary or fattening desserts are the exception, not the rule, in a Mediterranean meal. You can enjoy them a few times a week as special treats, but try making fresh fruit your regular dessert.

- **Drink in moderation.** No one needs to tell the Greeks to drink wine for their heart. They've been doing that for years. Moderate drinking – a glass of wine a day for women, and up to two a day for men – is a normal part of this diet.

   While heavy drinking is not a healthy habit, studies suggest moderate amounts of alcohol could reduce your risk of heart disease. If you're comfortable having a glass of wine with your meal, that's good news. However, don't feel you must start drinking.

It may sound like all Greek people do is eat, but regular exercise is an integral part of their health. Take a cue from them and combine physical activity with your new Mediterranean eating plan.

Dodge disease with the Asian diet

The humble life of a peasant may not be for you, but eating like one could save your heart and your health.

In the China-Cornell-Oxford Diet and Health Project, the largest study of its kind, researchers charted the eating habits of more than 10,000 Chinese, who happen to have amazingly low cholesterol levels and heart disease risk. Asians from other countries also enjoy uncommon protection from illnesses as diverse as cancer, heart disease, and obesity.

Experts are now piecing together a picture of the ideal Asian diet, one full of high-fiber, nutrient-rich plant foods and low in animal products and total fat – the kind that simple, rural Asian peasants eat.

Apparently, this diet works. Even the average high cholesterol in parts of Asia is about the same as the lowest range in the United States. Heart disease only accounts for about 15 percent of deaths there, a far cry from the more than 40 percent it claims in the United States.

Take the road to better health by filling your plate with these modest but magnificent foods.

- **Get on board with grains.** Rice, wheat, millet, corn, and barley – grains like these form the basis of most Asian diets. They are, however, less refined than the kind most Westerners eat, so they retain more natural fiber and other nutrients. Shop for unrefined rice to get a taste of good Asian health, and take a chance on exotic varieties like jasmine, basmati, or brown rice.

- **Add in the value of vegetables.** Exotic-sounding greens like bok choy, amaranth, bamboo shoots, and water spinach are second only to grains as key players in Asian diets. If you can't find these in your local store and don't have access to special markets, substitute more familiar, but equally healthy vegetables like broccoli, peppers, spinach, celery, carrots, and others. Spice them up for added flavor and a true taste of the Orient.

- **Make way for fruits.** Fresh fruits appear frequently at Asian meals. In fact, they're often served in place of desserts and sweets, a far better choice than the sugary, fatty treats Westerners often indulge in.

- **Don't forget legumes.** Asians understand the importance of the basic bean. They make soybeans into tofu, paste, noodles, sheets, and even eat them plain. Since people in this part of the world eat few animal foods, beans fill their protein requirements. In addition, they're loaded with fiber, phytoestrogens, and other nutrients.

  Whether you dip into unusual legumes like chickpeas, lentils, and mung beans, or stick to old standbys, just be sure you make them a regular part of your meals for an authentic Asian diet.

- **Nibble on nuts and seeds.** Pine nuts, almonds, walnuts, and cashews are just a few nuts you'll see gracing Asian dishes. Whether chopped and sprinkled over food, or crushed in sauces and dressings, a handful of nuts and seeds every day goes a long way toward total health. They are generally loaded with unsaturated fat, vitamin E, and ellagic acid, and help lower cholesterol, fight cancer, and boost your brainpower.

- **Fill your basket with fish.** These creatures of the sea are rich in omega-3 fatty acids and protein, plus have the added boon of being low in cholesterol. They're a healthier alternative to red meat and may be one reason people in Asia have such long lives and low cholesterol. The Japanese often serve fish raw, but if the idea makes you squeamish try it other Asian ways, for instance chunked up and cooked in stir-fries or soups.

- **Decide for yourself about dairy.** Daily milk, cheese, and yogurt simply aren't options for many people in Asia. Despite that, they enjoy unusually low rates of osteoporosis compared to Western countries where calcium-rich dairy foods are eaten much more often. Some experts think a plant-based diet could contribute to their amazing bone health.

- **Eat less red meat, poultry, and eggs.** The Asian diet includes less meat and, therefore, less animal protein than Western diets. Instead, Asians get most of their protein from plants like legumes, nuts, and seeds.

  This may mean a healthier heart and arteries in the long run. To eat the Asian way, try cutting back on red meat to one serving a month, and poultry and eggs to once a week.

- **Say farewell to sweets.** These treats are truly that in most Asian countries – a luxury. Fresh fruits more often grace the dessert table, providing a natural sugar fix. Stay away from sugary sweets and see if your taste buds take a liking to nutritious fruit goodies.

Low-sodium strategies save your heart

Over the ages, salt has proved its worth, particularly as a seasoning for dull foods. Unfortunately, the sodium in it may add to the growing problems with high blood pressure. Too much salt could even contribute to osteoporosis.

Your body only needs a small amount of sodium – around 500 milligrams (mg) each day – to run smoothly. That equals about one-fourth teaspoon of salt.

For your health's sake, experts recommend you limit sodium to less than 2,400 mg daily – about one teaspoon of salt. Unfortunately, most people ignore health warnings and eat between 3,100 and 6,000 mg of pure sodium every day – that's from one and one-half to three teaspoons of salt.

Only 20 to 30 percent of the sodium you get comes from adding table salt to your food. The rest comes from processed or prepackaged foods. Test yourself. If you practice these eating habits more than once a week, chances are you get too much salt.

- eat out

- snack on pretzels, potato chips, or other salty foods

- add table salt to your food

- eat prepackaged items like canned foods, frozen dinners, or processed meats and cheeses

Lowering your sodium might be especially challenging if you tend to rely on quick meals and snacks, but the life-saving results could be worth your effort.

You'll need to slash your salt if you take the DASH-Sodium challenge. People in the study who ate less than 1,200 mg of sodium each day saw the biggest drop in their blood pressure, but if that sounds too hard aim for a more moderate 2,400 mg.

Participants in the DASH-Sodium study used less salt in recipes, and ate low-salt versions of foods like bread and sauces, and unsalted snack foods like pretzels and nuts. Follow their lead, and try these other timely tips to shut down extra sodium and high blood pressure.

- **Load up on fruits and veggies.** In their natural, fresh form they're low in sodium and packed with potassium, a mineral that may help reduce blood pressure.

- **Season with other flavors.** Hide the saltshaker and try spices, herbs, vinegar, lemon, or lime juice instead. Be sure to use salt-free versions of seasoning blends.

- **Go easy on the sides.** Pickled foods, ketchup, mustard, horseradish, and barbecue sauces can carry lots of sodium. Treat even low-sodium versions of soy and teriyaki sauces like salt, and use them sparingly.

- **Avoid processed and prepackaged food.** TV dinners, instant rice and pasta mixes, salad dressings, and canned soups and broths are some of the biggest salt offenders. Try to eat fresh, unsalted, or low-sodium foods whenever you can.

- **Buy fresh or frozen fish, poultry, and meat.** These tend to have less salt than their canned and processed counterparts. The exceptions are cured meats like bacon and ham, which are usually loaded with salt.

- **Wash away salt.** You can cut the sodium in canned vegetables and meats up to 40 percent just by rinsing them with water before you eat them.

- **Read labels.** Products low in sodium often advertise that fact. Check the Nutrition Facts label, too, and look for foods with less than 5 percent – about 120 mg – of your maximum daily sodium allowance.

- **Drink plenty of water.** It's generally low in salt, and helps flush any excess out of your body. Check the labels on bottled water for their sodium content.

Most people have to worry about getting too much salt, not too little. Play it safe. Check with your doctor before changing your eating habits, and ask if it's all right to lower your sodium intake. If you exercise vigorously, slowly cut back on salt rather than ditching it all at once. This gives your body some time to adjust.

Sweet solutions check the sugar blues

Added sugar is a major health concern, providing lots of energy, or calories, but very few nutrients. Eating too much of it tends to edge nutritious foods out of your diet and contribute to both weight gain and tooth decay. Plus, foods with added sugar are often also loaded with saturated fat and cholesterol, prime suspects in many heart-related health problems.

Unfortunately, most people get far more sugar than they need in a day, mostly from processed, pre-packaged foods. Just 2 ounces of chocolate or a single 12-ounce cola may deliver more than 8 teaspoons of sugar, while half a cup of canned corn may pack another 3 teaspoons.

Because of natural variations in food, nutrient analyses can be off by up to 20 percent. So a 200-calorie food might actually have anywhere from 160 to 240 calories.

Sweeteners like honey and molasses fare little better, providing almost no nutrients but plenty of calories. In fact, teaspoon for teaspoon, honey harbors more calories than white sugar.

So what's a sweet tooth to do? First, get the full scoop on sugars from week eight of the Complete Nutrition eating plan described in the *Nutrition know-how* chapter. Then take a look at the following tips to limit added sugar and still satisfy your sweet cravings.

- **Drink wisely.** Quench your thirst with water rather than sugary sodas or fruit drinks. Add a dollop of juice for a hint of sweetness.

- **Meet the many faces of sugar.** Check ingredient labels for code words like corn sweetener, corn syrup, fruit juice concentrate, honey, syrup, invert sugar, malt syrup, molasses, table sugar, raw sugar, and brown sugar. Avoid foods that list a sugar among its first ingredients.

- **Sneak a peak at the Nutrition Facts label.** Compare the total sugars in similar products, and choose those with the least amount.

- **Crack the sugar code.** Ingredients ending in "-ose" are really sugars, too, like maltose, fructose, dextrose, sucrose, lactose, and glucose.

- **Pick unprocessed products.** Whole grains, fruits, and vegetables contain less added sugar than their processed, prepackaged counterparts. Many have a naturally sweet taste anyway.

- **Heat up for natural sweetness.** Make low-sugar dishes and serve them warm. This makes many foods taste sweeter.

- **Add flavor not sugar.** Cook with sweet-tasting spices like allspice, cinnamon, nutmeg, or cloves.

You don't necessarily need to restrict all added sugars in your diet unless your doctor or dietitian has recommended it. Most people can safely enjoy an occasional sweet treat. Notice how much sugar you eat every day, and start gradually cutting back if your sweet tooth is getting the best of your health.

Serve up feasts without the fat

You've heard all about how bad certain fats are for your body – especially your heart. Now it's time to take action.

Trimming fat from your diet is a good place to start, but it's not enough. You need to replace the unhealthy saturated and trans fats with the heart-loving family of mono- and polyunsaturated fats you read about in the *Nutrition know-how* chapter.

Begin making the switch with over 20 tasty and painless ways to eat less fat every day, plus tips to replace the harmful fats with healthy ones.

Aim for leaner, meaner meat

- Favor fish and poultry over red and processed meats. Occasionally eat beans, peas, lentils, and nuts instead of meat.

- Choose turkey over other types of luncheon meat since it's usually lower in fat.

- Limit the amount of liver, kidneys, and other organ meats you eat.

- Buy the leanest cuts of meat you can afford. Buy beef cuts with the words "loin" or "round" and pork with the words "loin" or "leg" in the name. Go with "choice" instead of "prime" meats, and choose those labeled "USDA Select."

- If you must eat processed meats like sausage, bacon, and cold cuts such as salami and bologna, pick low-fat versions.

Enjoy delicious low-fat dairy

- Switch to low-fat (1 percent) or nonfat (skim) milk instead of whole and reduced fat (2 percent) milk.

- Look for low-fat cheeses with less than 3 grams of fat per ounce. And cut down on full-fat, processed, and hard cheeses like American, cheddar, and brie.

- Use soft margarines. The softer they are, the less saturated fat they contain. Try tubs and tubes of margarine or vegetable oil spread.

- Buy margarine that lists a vegetable oil as its first ingredient. Steer clear of those made with hydrogenated or partially hydrogenated oils.

- Forget sour cream – use plain, low-fat yogurt instead.

Snack with satisfaction

- Read the ingredient lists and Nutrition Facts labels on snack foods and avoid those with saturated or hydrogenated fats and oils.

- Check the saturated fat, total fat, and cholesterol content on the Nutrition Facts label. Pick those with the fewest grams of fat, not necessarily the lowest percentages.

- Make fruit your dessert.

- Stay away from foods listing palm or coconut oils among the first ingredients. Look for those made with canola, corn, safflower, soybean, or sunflower oil instead.

- Replace fatty snack foods with whole, unprocessed fruits and vegetables rich in fiber and nutrients.

Learn the art of low-fat cooking

- Steam, bake, broil, poach, roast, or microwave food instead of breading and frying it.

- Remove the skin from poultry and trim the fat from meat before you cook it.

- After cooking ground meat, blot it with paper towels, then put it in a colander and rinse with hot water.

- Roast meat on a rack so fat drips away from it.

- Fry fish and other foods in olive or canola oil.

- Replace meat in your recipes with beans or tofu.

- Cook with egg whites or egg substitutes, and eat egg yolks and whole eggs in moderation.

- Substitute a little unsaturated olive or canola oil for solid fats like shortening, butter, lard, or margarine.

- Either skip foods with creamy sauces or make your own with low-fat ingredients.

- Use undiluted evaporated milk in place of cream in recipes.

- Refrigerate stews and soups before you eat them, and skim the solid fat from the top before reheating them.

- Jazz up the flavor but skip the fat by adding salsa, chili sauce, mustard, or vinegar to dishes.

- Top baked potatoes with a whipped mixture of lemon juice and low-fat cottage cheese.

The diet-disease connection

4

Slow the risk of Alzheimer's disease

You've learned that eating a nutritionally balanced diet may prevent or ease many health conditions. But if you suffer from a particular disease, you may need to focus on specific nutrients to really reap the benefits.

Alzheimer's disease (AD) is a mental disorder in which your brain cells gradually die, affecting your thinking, memory, behavior, and speech. Experts aren't sure exactly what causes this tragic disease, but they do know that eating the right foods, exercising, and learning new skills all seem to offer some protection. So while you can't predict the future, you can hedge your bets by adding these five helpful nutrients to your diet.

B vitamins fuel your brain

Brushing up on your B's could breathe life into your brain. Folate, thiamin, B6, and B12, in particular, are essential to your mental health, providing your brain the nutritional fuel it needs to stay active and alert.

B vitamins are also key in preventing Alzheimer's disease. The amino acid homocysteine has long been a culprit in heart disease and stroke. Now, new research by the National Institute on Aging shows that having high homocysteine levels nearly doubles your chances of AD – and the longer it stays high, the greater your risk. Folate, B6, and B12 ride to the rescue by reining in out-of-control homocysteine.

So put the brakes on aging with B vitamins. Leafy green vegetables, fortified grains, and legumes are terrific sources of both folate and B6, while low-fat or lean animal foods like meat and dairy products are your best bets for B12.

Slow AD with Vitamin E

While there's no cure for Alzheimer's disease, studies show an antioxidant like vitamin E might naturally slow its progress. Researchers tested vitamin E supplements and a popular Parkinson's drug called selegiline against a placebo. People with moderate AD who took selegiline or 2,000 international units (IU) of vitamin E each day were able to function and look after themselves seven months longer than those on the placebo.

The amount of vitamin E used in this study is far more than most people need in a day and could cause bleeding problems. Most doctors aren't ready to recommend treating AD with this much E. But you can safely get healthy amounts by eating a variety of seeds, nuts, vegetable oils, and leafy dark green vegetables. Sunflower seeds, wheat germ, and canola oil, in particular, are spectacular sources of vitamin E.

Boost your memory with beta carotene

An encouraging study showed that among 5,000 people between the ages of 55 and 95, those who fit the most beta carotene into their diets had the least trouble remembering, concentrating, and performing other mental tasks. The news is even better for Alzheimer's. A study at a university in Ohio shows a lifetime of eating colorful fruits and vegetables could lower your risk for AD. The smart secret? A potent package of antioxidants including beta carotene, vitamin A, and vitamin C in wholesome foods like tomatoes, carrots, and dark green and yellow vegetables.

Omega-3 fights inflammation

The same fatty acid that fights heart disease could lead the charge in fending off Alzheimer's. Some experts believe brain inflammation contributes to the slow descent into AD, so it makes sense that a natural anti-inflammatory like omega-3 could help you fight back.

Fatty fish are by far the best source of this nutrient, and most experts recommend eating two or more servings each week of salmon, mackerel, tuna, or other cold-water fish. Feeling green around the gills? Walnuts, flaxseed, and leafy dark green vegetables are fine omega-3 alternatives to fish. Fill the other half of the anti-inflammation equation by cutting back on omega-6 fatty acids in your diet. These can actually cause swelling and cancel out the benefit of omega-3. Skip the fried and fast foods as well as baked goods full of omega-6, and steer toward more balanced eating habits.

An easy way to get fatty fish into your diet is with a delicious salad like the one below. Try the five other healthy recipes in this chapter, and you'll reap the benefits of these anti-aging foods.

Alaska Salmon Waldorf Salad

1/2 cup light mayonnaise or salad dressing

1/4 cup plain nonfat yogurt

1/4 teaspoon lemon-pepper seasoning

1/2 teaspoon dried thyme

1/4 teaspoon salt

1 can (14 3/4-ounce) or 2 cans (7 1/2 ounces each) Alaska salmon, drained and chunked

2 ribs celery, diced (about 1 cup)

1 large apple, chopped (about 1 cup)

1/2 cup (2 ounces) broken walnuts

☆ In small bowl, blend mayonnaise, yogurt, lemon-pepper, thyme, and salt.

☆ In separate bowl, combine salmon, celery, apples, and walnuts.

☆ Stir dressing into salad.

Serves 3 to 4. Per serving: 353.7 calories; 21.2g total fat; 16.9g carbohydrate; 25.9g protein; 65mg cholesterol; 2.6g dietary fiber; 927.3mg sodium; 277.4mg calcium; 2.8g omega-3 fatty acids

Calcium: critical mineral for AD prevention

This mineral is crucial to strong bones, healthy blood pressure, good digestion, and even dodging certain kinds of cancer. Surprisingly, it may also protect your mind from memory loss as well as dementias such as Alzheimer's. Calcium plays an important role in helping your brain and nerve cells communicate. So while you're baking that fish and serving up fresh veggies, don't forget to make room for this critical mineral. Look for it in low-fat dairy products, calcium-fortified orange juice, and a variety of other foods like legumes and broccoli.

Fight asthma with foods

Asthma can attack at the worst times – when your allergies act up, during stressful periods, and even while you're exercising. Different people have different triggers, and some cases seem to come out of nowhere. During an attack, the muscles in your bronchi – the airways between your lungs and wind pipe – swell and spasm, making it difficult to breathe.

An attack can be frightening, but your condition doesn't have to leave you feeling helpless. Along with medication, your diet can make a difference in how you feel. If you find yourself out of breath, especially after exercising, these five nutrients may prove to be effective solutions.

Relieve congestion with vitamin C

Taking 1 to 2 grams of vitamin C a day helped people with asthma breathe easier in one small study. This could be because vitamin C is a natural antihistamine. You can find vitamin C in all sorts of tasty snacks like citrus fruits and juices, sweet red peppers, broccoli, brussels sprouts, and other brightly colored fruits and vegetables.

Lycopene: super EIA fighter

A dash of ketchup or a morning grapefruit could put a lid on asthma, particularly the kind that strikes while you're exercising. The difference is lycopene, a carotenoid that gives many fruits and vegetables their pinkish blush. People with exercise-induced asthma (EIA) took 30 milligrams (mg) of lycopene every day in one recent study. More than half of them felt their symptoms improve in just a week.

Although these asthma sufferers used supplements, you can get the same amount of lycopene from about a cup of tomato juice or half a cup of spaghetti sauce. Add a wedge of watermelon, a juicy pink grapefruit, or a slice of papaya for an extra dose of pink goodness. Here's more good news – many foods high in lycopene are also loaded with vitamin C, doubling your defenses.

Soothe spasms with magnesium

This mineral seems to soothe the muscle spasms in your bronchi that mark an attack. In fact, doctors have used one form of it – magnesium sulfate – to treat asthma. Mine this mineral from natural sources like seafood, nuts, legumes, and dark green vegetables. A handful of sunflower seeds, a side of pinto beans, or a sliced avocado can put you on your way to an asthma-free day. To get a hearty dose of magnesium, try this delicious soup full of beans and vegetables.

Garden Vegetable and Bean Soup

1 1/2 cups chopped onion

1 cup sliced celery

3 medium carrots, sliced

2 teaspoons minced garlic

1 tablespoon vegetable oil

2 cans (15 ounces each) Navy beans or Great Northern beans, or 3 cups cooked dry-packaged Navy or Great Northern beans, rinsed, drained, and divided

2 cans (14 1/2 ounces each) fat-free reduced-sodium chicken broth

2 cups broccoli florets

1/2 teaspoon dried rosemary leaves

1/4 teaspoon ground thyme leaves

1 cup salad spinach

Salt and pepper to taste

☆ Sauté onion, celery, carrots, and garlic in oil in large saucepan 3 to 4 minutes. Add 1 can beans, chicken broth, broccoli florets, and herbs to saucepan; heat to boiling. Reduce heat and simmer until broccoli is tender, 5 to 7 minutes.

☆ While soup is cooking, process remaining beans in food processor or mash until smooth. Stir puréed beans and spinach into soup; simmer until hot, about 2 minutes. Season to taste with salt and pepper.

Serves 6. Per serving (1 cup): 242 calories; 3g total fat; 40g carbohydrate; 16g protein; 0mg cholesterol; 3g dietary fiber; 884mg sodium;145mcg folate

Vitamin E edges out asthma

Too little vitamin E in your body seems to raise your risk for developing asthma, whereas upping your intake could give you an edge over this chronic illness. Try fending off future attacks by filling your plate with E-excellent foods like sweet potatoes, fortified cereals, wheat germ, sunflower seeds, and canola oil.

Breathe easier with selenium

People with asthma tend to be low on selenium, an antioxidant mineral that works a lot like vitamin E in your body. One study found that taking 100 micrograms (mcg) of sodium selenite, a selenium supplement, made it easier to breathe for people with asthma. Shop for whole grains, seafood, and meats like liver and kidneys before you head for the supplement aisle. They're the simple, natural path to more selenium.

Slash cancer risk with healthy diet

Cancer has no magic cure, but you can help protect your body from this dread disease by following a healthy diet and lifestyle. These simple steps also will help you avoid many other diseases – including heart disease and diabetes – that haunt the 50-plus age group.

Healthy food choices, plus exercise and not smoking or drinking alcohol, may prevent up to 70 percent of all cancers, experts say. If you're overweight, you're more likely to get certain types of cancer. Getting off the couch and lowering your fat intake is a good start, but the real key is a diet dominated by plant-based foods.

The National Cancer Institute's (NCI) dietary guidelines say to limit fat to 30 percent of your total calories, increase fiber to 20 to 30 grams a day, and include a variety of fruits and vegetables in your diet. By focusing on the superstar nutrients found in plant foods, you'll get the most anti-cancer punch from your diet.

Antioxidants attack free radicals

If just one cell in your body works improperly, it could create cancer. This possibility exists thanks to extra electrons called free radicals that invade your cells and make them unstable. What you need to fight back are antioxidants – powerful nutrients that cancel out free radicals before they have a chance to damage your cells. Foods loaded with antioxidants are important protectors against aging as well as cancer.

- Cruciferous vegetables like broccoli, cauliflower, cabbage, brussels sprouts, and kale are full of hard-hitting antioxidants such as vitamin C, beta carotene, and lutein. Also known as brassicas, these powerful foods contain phytochemicals that seem to protect your DNA from cancer-causing mutations. They may even curb the growth of harmful tumors. Brassicas are linked to reduced risk in studies of prostate, breast, lung, colon, stomach, brain, bladder, and other cancers.

- Bright red tomatoes are full of lycopene, a carotenoid antioxidant and a noted cancer crusher. It protects you against cancers of the colon, stomach, lung, esophagus, prostate, and throat. Also on the lycopene team are red grapefruit, guava, watermelon, and tomato-based products such as ketchup and spaghetti.

  The star of the future, however, may be a berry called the autumn olive, which has 17 times more lycopene than a tomato. Similar to a cranberry in taste and size, the autumn olive comes from a bush that survives in poor soil. It is sometimes considered a pest because it spreads when birds eat the berries and scatter the seeds. Watch for it, though, to show up as an ingredient in processed foods.

- Alliums – bulb vegetables that include garlic and onions – have lots of flavonoids that strike out free radicals and cancer. Garlic, with more than 100 chemical parts, may protect against cancer in your lungs, colon, kidneys, mouth, skin, and breasts. Crush garlic to release its full anti-cancer powers, and let it "rest" about 10 minutes before heating it.

- Don't forget green tea. It's loaded with antioxidants, and studies show it may help prevent almost every kind of cancer along with several other diseases. It may even boost the effects of chemotherapy treatment for existing cancers.

Fill up on folate to protect your genes

The B vitamin folate is an essential ingredient for making DNA. Without enough of this essential vitamin, you could end up with broken chromosomes, one risk factor for cancer. Folate helps maintain your genes to keep your cells from becoming cancerous. It's especially helpful in stopping colon cancer, and not having it increases your chances of getting cancer of the cervix, lung, esophagus, brain, pancreas, breast, and rectum. Get folate into your body by eating leafy green vegetables such as spinach and kale, beets, squash, enriched cereal, and beans.

Balance your body with omega-3

You need a balanced amount of both kinds of essential fatty acids – omega-3 and omega-6 – or you may put your body at risk for cancer. Researchers believe having more omega-6 than omega-3 in your body promotes the growth of cancerous tumors. Omega-6 fats are found in corn and soy oils, processed grains, and red meat. So you need to think twice about a diet of fried, fast, and processed food that gives you too much of this fatty acid. To get on an even keel, cut back on omega-6 fat and eat more omega-3s. Two servings a week of cold-water fish like salmon, tuna, herring, and mackerel is a good way to get back in balance. You can also get this "good" fat from flaxseed oil, walnuts, and green leafy vegetables.

Fix your diet with fiber

The NCI recommends you get 20 to 30 grams of fiber a day. Earlier research showed that a high-fiber diet helps prevent colon cancer, but newer research suggests it may not. It could be other nutrients in foods with fiber that provides the protection. For example, high-fiber, low-fat diets usually include lots of fruits and vegetables, which are linked to less cancer risk.

Still, fiber is an essential part of a healthy diet. Fiber adds bulk to your stool and hurries it through your large intestine, which limits the time cancer-causing agents spend in your body. Barley and oats, two outstanding sources of fiber, also work with organisms in your large bowel to form protective compounds. Wheat bran has phytic acid, which has antioxidant properties that may stop tumors.

When you eat highly processed, low-fiber foods, you get lower nutrition overall as well as a lack of regularity. So focus on eating more wholewheat bread, brown rice, and plenty of fruits and vegetables.

Selenium cancels out cancer threat

This trace mineral scores against a number of opponents, from asthma to yeast infections, and protects against skin and lung cancer in particular.

You can get selenium from beef, chicken, seafood, whole wheat, broccoli, celery, cucumbers, dairy products, and mushrooms. It is a soil-based nutrient, so the amount you get depends on the dirt where your food was grown. The northern plains generally produce the most selenium-rich food, but a normal diet of mostly unprocessed foods will provide all you need. Don't take selenium supplements without a doctor's supervision, though, because it is a toxic mineral, and too much is unsafe.

Slim down and eat right to avoid diabetes

You hear it over and over for heart disease, stroke, and cancer – lose weight and exercise if you want to stay alive. Well, add diabetes to the list. About three-fourths of all diabetics are overweight. And so many people with diabetes die from heart disease that the American Heart Association says it believes diabetes is a cardiovascular disease.

Diabetes mellitus results when your body doesn't process carbohydrates properly and you end up with too much glucose – blood sugar – in your system. But you can help control this condition with a diet that lets your body deal with food properly. Most sources of health advice, including the American Diabetes Association, favor a balanced high-carbohydrate, low-fat diet. Make sure it's rich in the following nutrients.

Vitamin C: top diabetes defender

This leading antioxidant is more than an offensive weapon against free radicals. It plays defense, too. Vitamin C helps control blood sugar levels, lowers blood cholesterol, and improves circulation. As an anti-oxidant, it helps protect you from the serious side effects of diabetes, such as blindness, amputation, heart disease, stroke, nerve damage, and kidney disease.

Get vitamin C from sweet red peppers, sweet potatoes, broccoli, and strawberries. Citrus fruits, another prime C source, have an added benefit for diabetics because the acid in those fruits slows down digestion and helps stabilize blood sugar. Vinegar works the same way. Three teaspoons of vinegar can lower blood sugar after a meal by 30 percent. Squeezing a lemon or lime into your water glass is a tasty way to do the same thing.

Omega-3 fights insulin resistance

You need this essential fatty acid to process insulin, and without it, you run the risk of developing insulin resistance, which is often your first stop on the road to diabetes. Unfortunately, most people don't get enough omega-3s. Cooking oils used today – corn, peanut, sesame, safflower – have mostly omega-6 oils, which are also essential fatty acids. But too much omega-6 will break down your immune system if you don't have the omega-3s to balance them out.

Fatty fish like salmon and mackerel; walnuts; and flaxseed are good sources of omega-3 oils, as is cod liver oil. Canola cooking oil has a good balance of both omega-3 and omega-6.

Rely on fiber to lower blood sugar

By slowing down the conversion of carbohydrates to glucose, fiber helps keep your blood sugar low. And your body responds to high-fiber carbs with less insulin than low fiber. Too much insulin can lead to weight gain and high blood pressure.

Lead off your day with a bran muffin or a bowl of bran cereal. Or have some oatmeal – oats contain beta glucan, which breaks down slowly in your digestive tract and keeps blood sugar down. Throughout the day, go for whole-wheat or rye breads and plenty of natural fruits and vegetables. Legumes – beans, peas, and lentils – have lots of fiber and are good substitutes for meat.

For a snack treat, try figs. They're tasty, high in fiber, low in fat, and full of antioxidants. For an extra advantage, take a little psyllium seed husk – the primary ingredient in Metamucil and similar products. A soluble fiber used mostly as a laxative, psyllium has shown amazing results in lowering blood sugar.

Add chromium for more sugar control

Chromium helps insulin move glucose out of your bloodstream and into your cells, thus lowering blood sugar. And taking chromium dramatically improved the severe shaking, blurred vision, sleepiness, and heavy sweating for a group of people with hypoglycemia. As with most minerals, you should ask your doctor before taking supplements. Get it naturally from dairy products, fish and seafood, liver, mushrooms, whole-grain products, fresh fruits, nuts, unpeeled potatoes and apples, and black pepper.

Biotin boosts digestion

A little-known B-vitamin – biotin – plays an important role in energy metabolism, growth, and the production of fatty acids and digestive enzymes. It helps digest fats and carbohydrates, which is important for diabetics. It also displays insulin-like activity in lowering blood sugar. In various tests, blood sugar levels in diabetics were cut in half, while insulin levels stayed the same. Biotin is found in peanut butter, liver, eggs, cereals, nuts, and legumes.

Blueprint for a healthy heart

Is artery disease lurking in your veins? If you have fatty plaque buildup, a clot in your arm or leg can gridlock your arteries just like a 5:00 traffic jam. And that situation puts you at risk for tissue damage or even a heart attack. Your doctor can do a simple test to determine if you have PAD – peripheral artery disease. He simply compares the blood pressure readings at your arm and ankle to assess your risk. Ask him about it today, especially if you have leg pain. If he does find PAD, heart medicines are not your only option. You have plenty of natural ways to control your cholesterol and thin your blood. Discover exactly which nutrients can help you improve your heart.

Omega-3 controls triglycerides

Cutting back on your fat intake too much can do your heart more harm then good. That's because your triglyceride levels can shoot up even as your good HDL cholesterol levels drop – if you try to maintain a diet with less than 20 percent fat. The key to heart health is not to cut all the fat out – it's to get the right kind of fat.

The omega-3 essential fatty acids in cold-water fish like tuna, salmon, and mackerel can bring down your LDL cholesterol numbers and keep your triglycerides under control. They will also keep your blood from getting sticky and clogging your arteries – both spelling health for your heart. In fact, if you add just one 3-ounce serving of fatty fish to your diet every week, you can cut your risk of a heart attack in half. And if you've already had a heart attack, just taking a fish oil supplement can lower the threat of a second attack by 10 percent. If you can't stomach seafood, you can get plenty of omega-3 fatty acids from flax and flaxseed oil or from fish oil supplements.

Add fiber to cut heart attack risk

Believe it or not, your breakfast cereal may save your life. With every 10 grams of fiber you add to your diet every day, you lower your chances of having a heart attack by 20 percent – about the same effect as dropping your cholesterol by 10 percent. Studies show that men who eat the most fiber generally have 55 percent less risk of a fatal heart attack than men with low-fiber diets. In fact, 21,000 men in Finland ate about 35 grams of fiber a day and watched the incidence of heart attack in their group drop by 25 percent compared to those who averaged only 16 grams a day.

Experts say you should strive for about 30 grams a day for best results. Whole grain cereals, vegetables, and fruit are all great sources of fiber. Try this simple and delicious barley recipe for a nutritious side dish that complements any meal.

Barley Pilaf

1 cup pearl barley
3 cups chicken or beef stock

☆ Mix broth and barley.
☆ Simmer 45 minutes or until tender.
☆ Salt to taste.
☆ Variations: Add shredded carrots and green pepper in the last few minutes of cooking. Serve with entree. If serving pork or poultry, chop 1 small apple, 1 small onion, and a stalk of celery, and add to the pilaf in the last five minutes of cooking. Season with thyme or sage.

Serves 6. Per serving (1/2 cup): 126 calories; 0.7g total fat; 26g carbohydrate; 4.7g protein; 0g cholesterol; 5.2g dietary fiber; 394.2mg sodium

---

Antioxidants: powerhouse artery cleaners

Get ready to ace heart attack 101 with vitamins A, C, and E. These tiny powerhouses are antioxidants – they stop cell destruction before it starts and help clear your arteries of plaque.

- **Vitamin A.** Beta carotene is a type of vitamin A found in brightly colored plant foods like apricots, carrots, pumpkins, and sweet potatoes. Studies show that if you get 15 to 20 milligrams (mg) of beta carotene a day, your risk of heart attack goes down 22 percent compared with those who get less than 6 mg.

- **Vitamin C.** If you have heart disease, you can help yourself live longer just by taking a simple aspirin daily. This is because it helps thin your blood and prevent clots. Vitamin C works in a similar way by strengthening the walls of your blood vessels and thinning your blood so your "highways" stay clear. Studies show it also helps raise HDL cholesterol levels. As little as 60 mg extra a day – the equivalent of an orange – can lower your heart disease risk. Strawberries, peaches, citrus fruits, and cantaloupe can all supply your daily C needs.

- **Vitamin E.** Protect your heart by getting plenty of vitamin E. It helps keep sticky plaque from building up in your arteries and also breaks up the plaque you already have so clots won't form. You may slash your heart attack risk by 37 percent if you're a man, or by 41 percent if you're a woman, just by adding 100 IU of vitamin E to your daily diet. You'll find vitamin E in sunflower seeds, canola oil, wheat germ, and nuts. Walnuts are especially good because they're rich in omega-3 fatty acids, which also thin your blood and help prevent clots.

- **Flavonoids.** Want to cut your heart attack risk by two thirds? Work plenty of tea, fruit, and vegetables into your diet. The flavonoids in foods like apples, green tea, and onions significantly reduced the risk of heart disease in a study group in Holland. Apples and apple juice may prevent bad LDL from turning into sticky plaque. And one study found that drinking a 10- to 12-oz glass of purple grape juice each day may reduce blood clotting by 39 percent.

  Green tea has flavonoids called catechins that slash cholesterol and triglyceride numbers significantly. Drink several cups a day for best results. Black tea helps open up your blood vessels, which heart disease constricts. Three cups a day may keep your arteries free of cholesterol traffic jams.

- Garlic and onions protect you not only from heart disease, but also from cancer and premature aging.

> **Do not exercise after drinking coffee, especially if you have high blood pressure. It shrinks your blood vessels and can cause a heart attack while you work out.**

The flavonoids in garlic keep your arteries soft and flexible and thin your blood so it doesn't clump. Add one crushed and lightly sautéed clove to your meals every day. Sliced red and yellow onions also protect your heart. Cook them in place of salt to help season your dinner and fight high blood pressure.

Minerals guarantee a regular heartbeat

You need the right amount of magnesium and potassium to keep the electrical activity of your heart regular. The potassium in bananas can help lower your blood pressure and protect your heart. Spinach, beans, and a baked potato with skin provide you with magnesium – and long-term protection from artery spasms, irregular heartbeat, and high cholesterol. Okra and persimmons are rich in both, so why not be adventurous and add these unusual foods to your shopping list?

Eat to defeat macular degeneration

Macular degeneration is the leading cause of blindness in people over age 65. Sometimes called age-related macular degeneration or AMD, this condition affects the retina of your eye and takes away the central part of your vision.

Most people have dry AMD, which generally causes less serious vision loss. It's not even painful. Fine details just gradually become harder to make out as your central vision blurs or distorts. Of those with macular degeneration, only 10 percent have wet AMD – the painful kind that may cause permanent vision loss within weeks or days. So far, medications and surgeries for AMD have had only limited success.

You're at higher than average risk for AMD if you're far-sighted, smoke, have light-colored eyes, have spent a lot of time in the sun, and have a family history of AMD or heart disease. Yet scientists suggest that eating right may help you shield your eyes from AMD before it starts. Recruit these nutritional allies to help you see well into your future.

Carotenoids slash your risk

The same carotenoids that bring vivid color to foods may help keep your sight vivid into old age. In fact, research found that people who ate more carotenoids slashed their risk of developing AMD by 43 percent. Eating spinach and collard greens seemed especially helpful – perhaps because they're both rich in the carotenoids lutein and zeaxanthin.

Your eye's retina is extremely rich in lutein and zeaxanthin, too. Experts believe these antioxidants defend the eye against light damage while supporting the blood vessels to the retina. Eat to raise your body's levels of lutein and zeaxanthin, and you may keep your retina strong, efficient, and better equipped to fight the damage that may cause AMD. Try lutein-loaded corn or orange peppers full of zeaxanthin. Add more of both carotenoids by eating kiwi, red seedless grapes, kale, or zucchini.

Beta carotene and lycopene are carotenoids that may also help. Get lycopene from anything made with tomato paste or tomato sauce. Serve up beta carotene from sweet potatoes, cantaloupes, pumpkins, or carrots.

Omega-3 repairs retinal damage

To protect your eyes, go fish! A special omega-3 fatty acid in fish called docosahexaenoic acid (DHA) also rests in the retina. DHA may even protect and restore retinal cell membranes, helping to repair damage there. Fish may also help by keeping your arteries clean.

Studies verify that fish may be valuable to your vision. One study found that eating more fish – especially tuna – significantly slices your odds of AMD. Another study discovered that eating fish once a week reeled in the most protection.

Fatty fish like salmon, mackerel, herring, and tuna offer the most omega-3, but all seafood contains some. For fish-free omega-3, eat flaxseed, walnuts, and mustard, turnip, or collard greens. Dark green leafy vegetables like spinach, Swiss chard, arugula, and kale also give you some omega-3.

Just remember that if you eat unhealthy fats, the help from omega-3 fats could become "the one that got away." According to the Massachusetts Eye and Ear study, fish and omega-3 fatty acids seem to lower the risk for AMD, but only if your diet does not include much linoleic acid (omega-6 fatty acids). So pass up margarine, corn oil, and soybean oil, and eat more fish instead.

Combat AMD with vitamin C

Lutein, zeaxanthin, and omega-3s aren't the only antioxidants shining in your eyes. Healthy eyes have a high concentration of antioxidant vitamin

C, too. One study seems to suggest that distressed eyes could benefit from more vitamin C. The National Eye Institute's Age-Related Eye Disease Study (AREDS) showed that high doses of antioxidant vitamins plus zinc helped slow AMD before it reached an advanced stage. Each day, people in the six-year study took 500 milligrams (mg) of vitamin C, 15 mg of beta carotene, vitamin E, and 80 mg of zinc. Those with intermediate macular degeneration cut their risk for advanced AMD by 25 percent. They also slashed their odds of vision loss by 19 percent.

Although it's best to get your nutrients from whole foods, you may need supplements to get enough antioxidants to combat AMD. But get as much vitamin C from food as you can. Eat red or green peppers or citrus fruits for the vitamin C that may help you see.

Add vitamin E to protect your eyes

Healthy eyes have plenty of vitamin E, too. To aid their ailing eyes, volunteers in the AREDS study took 400 international units (IU) of vitamin E along with their vitamin C each day. Vitamin E and vitamin C help each other do their jobs – and end up protecting your retinas from the free radical damage that may lead to eye disease. Although you may need to get extra antioxidant power from supplements, you can absorb lots of vitamins C and E from brightly colored vegetables and fruits, like apricots, carrots, and red and green peppers. Dark, leafy greens are also good ways to slip vitamin C and vitamin E into your diet. For extra E, eat nuts, seeds, wheat germ, and vegetable oils.

Zinc: potent free-radical fighter

Zinc is especially concentrated in your retinas where it fights free radicals and helps in other ways to protect your eyes from AMD. Researchers have found a connection between low levels of zinc and a higher risk of AMD. In fact, you may have noticed that zinc was part of the AREDS study combination that helped fight advanced AMD and vision loss.

What's more, some doctors treat macular degeneration with zinc supplements. If you have AMD and think these might help you, check with your doctor first. It's easy to get too much zinc from supplements.

Older adults can sometimes be deficient in this mineral, so try to focus on eating foods like oysters, crabmeat, beefsteak, poultry, soybeans, enriched cereal, and yogurt. Your body absorbs zinc best from meat, but vegetarians who eat whole-grain breads leavened with yeast should get enough.

Winning ways to overcome osteoarthritis

What do Nolan Ryan, Joe Namath, and Dorothy Hamill have in common? They are all great athletes, and they all cope with osteoarthritis (OA). It's normal for cartilage and bones to deteriorate a little with daily wear and tear. But when the cartilage gets inflamed and breaks down completely, the bones rub against each other. This causes the serious pain and stiffness associated with osteoarthritis.

Exercise and good nutrition can help you overcome flare-ups of arthritis. Exercise strengthens the muscles holding your joints together and takes the pressure off your bones. Good nutrition can fight the inflammation that causes arthritis in the first place.

Ease joint pain with vitamin B

If you notice someone with large, swollen knuckles, you're probably looking at a victim of arthritis. Now, experts in Missouri think vitamin B can help you avoid such painful, unsightly joints. They gave a mix of two B vitamins, folic acid and vitamin B12, to people with arthritis in their hands. Those that took the B vitamins had far less pain and tenderness in their joints. Their grip also improved – about as much as it did while taking NSAIDs (non-steroidal anti-inflammatory drugs).

B vitamins are plentiful in foods like liver, beans, and greens. Participants in this study took relatively large doses – about 6,400 micrograms a day, which translates into a lot of greens. Talk to your doctor if you would rather take a supplement. This vitamin may not erase your pain completely, but a simple acetaminophen (Tylenol) should help with the rest.

Vitamin C fights inflammation

Most of your daily activities hinge on your knees – and vitamin C can protect them from falling apart. Vitamin C is an antioxidant that fights inflammation in your joints. It can also repair and cushion them with strong and healthy cartilage, even providing some pain relief. In one study, arthritis in people with low levels of vitamin C progressed three times faster than those with the highest amount of Cs in their system. You can get all the benefits of vitamin C from a diet rich in colorful fruit and vegetables like oranges, strawberries, and red peppers. Try another pepper – a chili pepper – for a day's supply of vitamin C as well as beta carotene. It not only helps your joints but soothes sore muscles, too.

Protect your cartilage with vitamin D

Your body cannot absorb calcium or build bones properly without vitamin D. Doctors who researched the role of vitamin D in osteoarthritis think the vitamin may protect the cartilage in your joints. They think it's also possible vitamin D may actually keep the bones of your joints intact. It's not hard to get vitamin D naturally, either. Just sit out in the sun for five minutes two or three times a week, and you'll get plenty of this mighty vitamin. When sunlight is scarce, refuel with fortified dairy foods, seafood and eggs. With your stores of D full, your arthritis is three times less likely to get worse, one study shows.

Soothe your aches with spicy ginger

A group of OA sufferers in Denmark ate 5 grams of fresh ginger a day, and three quarters of them reported significant relief from the achy pain and swelling of arthritis. In fact, the more ginger they ate, the better they felt. Researchers think ginger may work as a natural anti-inflammatory, reducing the redness, pain, and swelling that often accompanies arthritis.

If you want to try it for yourself, chop up a little fresh ginger each day, and lightly sauté it. Or add the dried root to your food for the same effect. If it helps relieve your pain, you may be able to cut back on your NSAIDs, which can produce serious side effects in some people. For an easy, tasty way to use fresh ginger, try the recipe on the next page.

Glucosamine: the miracle joint preserver

Studies have shown that at least one arthritis supplement may work, particularly in relieving knee pain. Glucosamine is naturally found in your body and is a major building block of the cartilage that cushions your joints and keeps your bones from rubbing together. If you don't have enough in your body, your cartilage breaks down. By taking a supplement of glucosamine extracted from clamshells you may help repair that damage. Research shows these little pills may cut the pain of OA and preserve your joints.

While it may take a couple of months to see results, glucosamine won't bother your insides like NSAIDs. The usual dosage is 500 mg three times a day, but be sure to check with your doctor before starting this supplement. He can make sure it's an appropriate treatment that won't interfere with your other medications.

Roasted Honey-Ginger Carrots

1 tablespoon sesame oil
1 tablespoon honey
1 tablespoon fresh ginger, grated
2 cloves garlic, minced
1 teaspoon soy sauce
1 pound baby carrots

☆ Combine the sesame oil, honey, ginger, garlic, and soy sauce, and mix well. Pour over the carrots and toss to coat.

☆ Place carrots in pie plate or casserole dish. Roast uncovered at 375 degrees for 30 minutes or until tender.

☆ Remove to serving platter, drizzle remaining glaze over carrots, and serve hot.

Serves 4. Per serving: 93 calories; 4g total fat; 14.4g carbohydrate; 1.2g protein; 0g cholesterol; 2.1g dietary fiber; 124.14mg sodium

Diet defense for osteoporosis

Osteoporosis can be so silent you don't even know you have it – until a broken bone or fracture lands you in the hospital. This disease usually develops because your diet doesn't include enough calcium and other bone-building nutrients. Without proper nutrition you could end up with weak, frail bones in your later years, and once you have osteoporosis, even mild stress on your bones can lead to injuries.

Luckily, this disease is a breeze to prevent and treat with proper nutrition. "The most important thing a woman can do to prevent osteoporosis is good nutrition and exercise habits, ideally before puberty," says Dr. Connie Weaver, head of Purdue University's Department of Food and Nutrition. But the same advice is important after menopause as well, she adds. So stand strong, not stooped, with these easy ways to keep your bones from becoming brittle.

Make calcium a top priority

The amount of calcium you get during your first 40 years of life can strongly predict your later risk for osteoporosis, so you should make this mineral a priority early on. Unfortunately, 75 percent of women under age 35 don't get enough daily calcium.

If you think you're one of them, don't give up hope. It's never too late to start protecting your bones. Men and women over age 51 should both aim to get 1,200 milligrams (mg) of calcium each day whether from dairy foods like low-fat milk and yogurt, vegetables such as collards and kale, or fish like bony salmon and sardines. Breakfast cereals and enriched orange juice also rate high in calcium.

Your body can only absorb about 500 mg of this mineral in a sitting. Instead of cramming all of your calcium into one meal, try to spread it throughout the day. And don't let up on your calcium crusade. Any gains you make in bone strength are lost within a year if you stop getting enough. For a delicious dose of calcium, whip up a fresh fruit smoothie like the one on the next page.

Add vitamin D for double protection

Upping your calcium alone may not stop osteoporosis. You actually need other vitamins and minerals to help you get the most from this important mineral. Vitamin D plays a big role in how much calcium your body absorbs. In fact, low levels of D go hand-in-hand with weaker, more fragile bones.

You'll be glad to know some of the same foods recommended for calcium like fortified milk, cereals, salmon, and sardines are also packed with vitamin D. Surprisingly, though, sunlight is one of the best sources of this nutrient. Your skin naturally turns sunshine into vitamin D, so a few minutes of walking or gardening outdoors could actually help build your bones.

As you age, your skin tends to make less D from its sunshine time, and sunscreens block the rays even more. But don't trade a painful burn for strong bones. Instead, rely on a variety of sources – foods as well as sunlight – to get 400 to 800 International Units (IU) of vitamin D each day.

Strawberry-Orange Smoothies

1 pint basket California strawberries, washed and stemmed

1 1/4 cups low-fat milk

2/3 cup unflavored low-fat yogurt

2 1/2 tablespoons frozen orange juice concentrate

2 tablespoons honey

4 ice cubes

☆ Combine all ingredients in container of electric blender. Blend until smooth.

☆ Pour into four 8-ounce glasses. Garnish with orange wheels, if desired. Serve with straws.

Serves 4. Per serving: 140 calories, 2g total fat, 25g carbohydrate; 5g protein; 8mg cholesterol; 2g dietary fiber; 70mg sodium; 185.8mg calcium

Vitamin K slashes fracture risk

It may not be the most well-known vitamin, but K is making medical news. Researchers at Harvard Medical School have linked vitamin K deficiencies to brittle bones and high fracture rates.

The two foods most likely to ride to your rescue are iceberg lettuce and broccoli. This humble lettuce may not be as exciting as its exotic counterparts, but it's still tops for taking care of your bones. Women in the Harvard study who ate a cup of iceberg lettuce – about 146 micrograms (mcg) of vitamin K – each day dropped their risk of hip fracture by 45 percent.

Broccoli lovers could also be in for a treat. Out of more than 1,000 women over age 67, those who ate broccoli at least three times a week had the fewest hip fractures and the least bone loss, a recent study showed. Experts think broccoli's rich vitamin-K content is the key. Toss a bone-saving salad with iceberg lettuce, fresh broccoli, cauliflower, and parsley to kick off your game against osteoporosis.

Choose bone-strengthening minerals

Potassium and magnesium are big players in heart health, but they're also essential for strong bones. Like vitamin D, they help your body make use of calcium. Researchers found out how important these minerals were when a group of men raised their bone density and lowered their risk of breaking a hip with every extra serving of fruits or vegetables they ate each day. So while you're taking in other nutrients, be sure to include foods loaded with magnesium like nuts, beans, oranges, and dark leafy greens, as well as fish, avocados, dried figs, bananas, and prunes for potassium. You'll do your heart and your hips a favor.

Focus on amazing antioxidants

Skip the bone-robbing coffees and colas when snack time rolls around. Instead, take notes from the British and take a cup of tea. Antioxidants – particularly the flavonoids – in black and green tea seem to protect your bones from osteoporosis. Scientists discovered that British women who drink tea have stronger bones than those who don't. You could pour milk in your tea for an added calcium boost, but don't drink more than 32 ounces of caffeinated tea a day. Caffeine actually weakens your bones, canceling out the tea-totaling benefits.

Nutritional ways to cope with RA

Rheumatoid arthritis (RA) is different from osteoarthritis although it may hurt just as much. RA starts when your immune system goes haywire and white blood cells – whose normal job is to fight harmful bacteria – start attacking the soft tissue in your joints. The result is painful and swollen joints – the same as in osteoarthritis, which is caused by wear and tear on those same cartilage tissues.

Left untreated, RA can permanently damage bone and cartilage and even spread to internal organs like your heart and lungs. People with RA are three times more likely to suffer heart attack or stroke, so see a rheumatologist and get treatment early to prevent the disease from getting ahead of you.

The right foods and regular exercise help smooth out the effects of RA, which is usually treated with nonsteroidal anti-inflammatory drugs (NSAIDs) or other strong medications that can have serious side effects.

High-fiber, low-fat foods help manage your weight, which is important because extra pounds put extra strain on your aching joints. And at least one study shows that a strict vegetarian, gluten-free diet may ease your arthritis pain. Make sure you get enough of these nutrients to give your body plenty of ammunition to battle this disease.

Omega-3 controls inflammation

Omega-3 fatty acids have anti-inflammatory powers that may soothe your achy joints enough to allow you to cut back on your NSAIDs, especially if you also take vitamin E. It works on RA by controlling cytokines, molecules that have to do with inflammation. Omega-3 also zaps triglycerides – villains in both RA and heart disease – and may even lower blood pressure.

You get the most omega-3 from fatty fish like salmon, tuna, and mackerel, and it's best to prepare it by boiling or baking. Research has found that fried fish doesn't offer any relief for arthritis. The next-best source of omega-3 is flaxseed oil. It has an earthy, fishy taste, so try disguising it on salads or vegetables. Or grind whole flaxseeds, and sprinkle them on hot or cold cereals, salads, or in baked goods.

Antioxidants knock out free radicals

Rheumatoid arthritis sufferers tend to be overloaded with free radicals and low on antioxidants. Scientists think free radicals and arthritis pain may be linked and that antioxidants may be able to knock them both out.

Vitamin E, selenium, and resveratrol seem to be particularly helpful against RA. Resveratrol comes from peanuts and grapes. Seafood, mushrooms, and whole wheat are good sources of selenium. Get vitamin E from wheat germ oil, sunflower seeds, avocados, and dry roasted peanuts. Pumpkin seed oil – used for cooking and in salad dressings – is rich in both vitamin E and selenium, as well as other antioxidants and omega-3 fatty acids, making it a potent inflammation fighter.

Curcumin: top pain-fighting phytochemical

The Arthritis Foundation lists turmeric and ginger as alternate therapies for RA. Curcumin, a powerful phytochemical with pain-fighting powers, is most likely the reason these spices offer relief. Experts say turmeric's effect on pain and swelling may equal that of NSAIDs, but without the side effects. Turmeric is the main spice in curry powder, so it's easy to get, especially if you like Indian or Thai food. Ginger also offers pain relief and can be eaten raw or candied, made into a tea, or taken in pill form. (See *Winning ways to overcome osteoarthritis* for an easy and delicious ginger recipe.) Talk to your doctor about taking ginger, though, if you regularly take NSAIDs or blood-thinning medication. It can interfere with blood clotting, causing you to bruise or bleed.

Count on fatty acids to reduce swelling

The monounsaturated fatty acids (MUFAs) in olive oil appear to work like omega-3 fatty acids by helping to reduce joint swelling. MUFAs are found in other oils, too, but olive oil is preferred because it also contains vitamin E and other powerful antioxidants that help combat the achy joints of arthritis. Plus it has no cholesterol and no "bad" saturated fats. Avocados and most nuts have lots of MUFAs, and so does a nut that's not a nut. The peanut is actually a legume, but it's a lot like olive oil because it has no cholesterol and is high in antioxidant power. A handful of nuts every day or a few teaspoons of olive oil may help give you the relief you need.

Water: a soothing cushion for your joints

An easy path to possible arthritis relief is simply to drink plenty of water every day. It lubricates and cushions your joints and is a key ingredient in the cartilage that holds your joints together. Water also helps arthritis through hydrotherapy. Water in a spa or pool that is between 85 and 98 degrees Fahrenheit gets your circulation going and keeps you limber. Water provides more resistance to exercise, so your muscles get a better workout. At the same time, it supports your limbs, causing less stress on your sore joints.

Secrets to avoiding stroke

Imagine what would happen if all the oxygen disappeared from the atmosphere – you wouldn't be able to breathe. The same thing happens to your brain when a blood clot keeps fresh oxygen from reaching thought-central – your cells start dying. This is called an ischemic stroke. If a blood vessel bursts, and your oxygen supply stops because it is being diverted somewhere else, the stroke is called hemorrhagic. According to the American Stroke Association, someone in America has a stroke every 53 seconds.

But you don't have to be a statistic. Even if your risk is high because of genetics, lifestyle, or stress, you can lower it with proper nutrition and exercise. Here are some guidelines to help you along.

Cut stroke risk with omega-3

Eat twice the fish and have half as many strokes. That's the newest finding from researchers at Harvard Medical School and the University of Miami School of Medicine. At the end of a 14-year study they concluded that the more fatty fish you eat, the better your chances of living stroke-free. Why fish? They're a good source of omega-3 fatty acids, a powerful anti-clotting compound.

Ditch deep-fried food. It's the #1 food to avoid to keep cholesterol under control and bring stroke risk down.

So make like an Eskimo and eat about 5 ounces of anchovies, herring, mackerel, mullet, salmon, trout, tuna, or whitefish each week to halve your risk of stroke. But don't go overboard – more than two fish a day can thin your blood too much, which may cause a bleeding stroke.

Alpha-linolenic fatty acids – a kind of omega-3 fat found in nuts and oils like canola, olive, and soy – may also cut your risk of suffering a stroke. A study in California found that for every 0.13 percent increase of this acid in your blood, the danger of suffering a stroke drops 37 percent.

Switch your generic vegetable oil with one of these oils, and substitute some nuts for a meat protein. Your heart will reap the benefits.

Calcium fights high blood pressure

Stop worrying and drink more milk – you just may help yourself avoid a stroke. A 22-year study showed that people who drank two cups of milk a day had half as many strokes as those who didn't drink milk. That's because the calcium in milk helps control your blood pressure, which lowers your risk. Make sure you drink the low-fat variety to protect your arteries from fat buildup. A calcium supplement is not as effective – there's just something about milk that makes it a first-rate stroke-buster.

Avoid potential threat with potassium

One Harvard professor is going bananas. He found out that high levels of potassium in bananas and other foods like apricots, avocado, figs, beans, and cantaloupes can decrease the threat of stroke. In fact, those with the most potassium in their system have 38 percent fewer strokes – perhaps because potassium helps lower your blood pressure. Just like milk, potassium from whole foods works best. Try to get it from your diet, not from supplements.

Fiber shakes off stubborn cholesterol

Seventy-five thousand women can't be wrong. In the famous Nurses Health Study in Boston, researchers found that those who ate lots of whole grains cut their chances of having an ischemic stroke almost in half. In a different study, men who ate 29 grams of fiber a day were 43 percent less likely to have a stroke, compared to those who ate only half that much. Fiber is famous for lowering both your blood pressure and your cholesterol. You can get your entire daily fiber quota from just one cup of pearl barley, two cups of cooked lima beans, or three cups of sweetened raspberries. All whole grains and beans, and most fruit and vegetables, are high in fiber.

To fully benefit from these all-stars, don't salt your food before you eat it. The American Heart Association recommends you keep your salt intake under 2.4 grams a day, about one teaspoonful. Most of this you already get from prepackaged or prepared foods.

Be smart and take B vitamins

Studies have shown B vitamins can help lower your risk of suffering a heart attack or stroke by controlling homocysteine levels. This substance, a by-product of protein metabolism, can damage and narrow your arteries. Even young people are at risk of damage from high levels of homocysteine. In a study on women ages 15 to 44, those with the highest levels of homocysteine were twice as likely to suffer a stroke as those having lower levels.

B vitamins also may come to the rescue after a stroke. Researchers studied 50 stroke survivors for three months. They found that the group taking a B-vitamin supplement had lower levels of homocysteine and thrombomodulin, a chemical indicator of blood vessel damage, than those not taking B vitamins.

An herbal solution to varicose vei

Do your legs itch and swell as the day wears on? ▪▪▪▪
may be pooling in your ankles because of faulty valves.
But you may be able to throw away your compression
stockings if you try horse chestnut instead. After two
weeks of taking this herbal extract, the swelling and leg
pain in your calves and ankles should lessen. Just make
sure there are at least 100 to 150 milligrams of escin,
the active ingredient, in each dose.

5 paths to more radiant skin

Go to your favorite drug store or department store, and you'll find no
shortage of expensive creams and lotions that promise you softer,
younger-looking skin. Yet good nutrition and healthy eating may be far
more important than slathering on expensive potions. Before you spend
a fortune on skin products, try these nutritional all-stars. Radiant skin
could be yours in no time.

Include omega-3 for baby-soft skin

Just as parched flowers need water, your skin needs soothing oils to keep
it soft and youthful. Cold-water fatty fish contain enriching omega-3 fatty
acids – a nutritious fat that may protect skin and fight inflammation. To
let your skin soak up the most omega-3s, eat fish such as Alaskan salmon,
mackerel, tuna, or sardines.

Yet keep in mind that some fish may be polluted with mercury from their
environment. Most people don't eat enough fish to be at high risk of mercury poisoning, but this metal can cause brain damage and interfere with
the development of unborn and young children. To play it safe, adults
may want to eat only one can of white tuna per week or two cans of light
tuna. Young children should probably have no more than one tuna fish
sandwich each week. When you choose mackerel, stick to Northern,
Atlantic, or Spanish mackerel that may have lower mercury risk. Farm-
raised fish could be another good way to play it safe.

.llubbers may prefer their omega-3 from flaxseed, walnuts, and mus-
rd, turnip, or collard greens. Dark green leafy vegetables like spinach,
Swiss chard, arugula, and kale also give you some omega-3.

Here's something else to consider. The omega-6 in fried foods, fast foods,
and baked goods can cancel out the skin-helping effects of omega-3. To
get omega-3's full benefits, cut back on omega-6 fatty acids in your diet.

Vitamin E: your skin's guardian angel

Too much sunlight does more than just burn and dry your skin. It may
also cause the kind of skin damage that ushers in wrinkles and skin aging.
Sunscreen is a good first defense against the harsh light of day, but why
stop there? Add in vitamin E's antioxidant power to guard your skin.
Although ultraviolet light from the sun can lead to free radicals that rav-
age your skin cells, vitamin E's antioxidants disarm free radicals like a
professional bomb squad. Scientists suggest that fending off free-radical
damage could mean healthier skin that stays young longer.

You can get vitamin E from what germ oil, sunflower seeds, almonds,
and turnip greens. And if you get your vitamin E from olive oil, you may
get some bonus protection against wrinkle-promoting sun damage. Not
only does olive oil arm you with its vitamin E, its monounsaturated fats
may help your skin cells resist sun damage even more powerfully.

And here's a tip. Japanese research with mice suggests you may limit skin
cell damage by rubbing extra virgin olive oil on your skin after coming in
from the sun. Just remember, only extra virgin olive oil will work, and
only after you're done with the sun.

Vitamin A: an A-1 skin protector

Protecting skin is one of vitamin A's main jobs, so it's important to make
sure you're getting as much as you need. If your cells can't get enough
vitamin A, some of them are replaced by cells that secrete keratin – the
substance that makes your hair and fingernails tough. It also makes your
skin dry, hard, and cracked like salt flats in the desert.

Fortunately, you have two easy ways to guard against this. First, get vitamin A from foods like meat and dairy products. Secondly, let your body
convert the beta carotene from fruits and vegetables into vitamin A. For
more beta carotene per bite, choose brightly colored produce like carrots, sweet potatoes, spinach, cantaloupe, apricots, and broccoli.

Banish wrinkles with vitamin C

Vitamin C helps make and maintain collagen, which forms the basis of connective tissue in your skin. This helps keep your skin from sagging and wrinkles from forming. Collagen also forms scar tissue to help heal wounds and supports tiny blood vessels to prevent bruises.

To keep your skin looking supple and young, get plenty of vitamin C in your diet. Good sources include sweet red peppers, citrus fruits, green peppers, and strawberries. Try filling the fruit tarts below with strawberries, tangerines, kiwi fruit, mangoes, or guava for a big boost of vitamin C.

Fresh Fruit Tarts

1/2 cup nonfat or low-fat sour cream

2 tablespoons confectioners' sugar

1 teaspoon chopped fresh mint or 1/4 teaspoon dried mint, crushed

4-ounce package single-serve graham cracker crusts (6 small crusts)

1 cup assorted cut-up fresh fruit

1/3 cup nonfat or low-fat lemon yogurt

☆ In a small bowl, stir together sour cream, confectioners' sugar, and mint. Spoon into graham cracker crusts. Arrange fruit over sour cream mixture.

☆ Serve immediately, or cover and refrigerate until serving time.

☆ Just before serving, stir yogurt and drizzle over fruit.

Serves 6. Per serving: 139 calories; 6g total fat; 19g carbohydrate; 3g protein; 4mg cholesterol; 82mg sodium

Nourish your cells with water

In the windswept chill of winter or the parching heat of summer, your skin can become dry and your lips chapped. Drink lots of clear, sparkling water to help keep your lips and skin dewy and comfortable. Water also teams up with vitamins to help your skin stay soft and smooth.

Don't wait until you feel thirsty to drink water. Your thirst, especially as you get older, may not be a reliable gauge of your body's need. You could be two cups low before you feel it. So rehydrate your skin every chance you get. After all, most people need 8 to 12 cups a day, and you may be pleasantly surprised at the results.

Easy ways to look your best

Whether you're going to a business meeting or spending an evening relaxing, you want to look your best. Healthy teeth, beautiful nails, and lustrous, shiny hair add to a polished appearance no matter what the occasion. Focus on getting enough of these nutrients, and you'll stack the beauty odds in your favor.

Calcium: your teeth's best friend

When you go out to meet old friends – or make new ones – you'd like to greet them with fresh breath and a mega-watt smile. Calcium may help you do both.

It's no secret that calcium forges strong teeth and helps you keep them that way. Yet you might be surprised to discover that some calcium-rich foods zap bad breath. Both yogurt and buttermilk bring you friendly lactobacillus – active cultures of bacteria that make it tough for odor-causing bacteria to grow. When buying yogurt, check for a label that promises active cultures. You may be glad you did.

Of course, you're not limited to buttermilk and yogurt. Power up with 1,200 milligrams (mg) of calcium a day if you're over 50 – or at least 1,000 mg if you haven't reached 50 yet. Get calcium from low-fat dairy products, green leafy vegetables, broccoli, cabbage, cauliflower, or nuts.

Fluoride brightens your smile

Fluoride is another teeth-building mineral. Most towns and cities add fluoride to their water supplies, so drinking good old-fashioned tap water may help your grin. But if you drink well water, bottled water, or purified water, you may be missing out. That's because these water sources can be short on fluoride.

Make up the loss with tea, apples, eggs, and seafood. In fact, green tea may also guard your mouth by curbing the growth of bacteria that cause cavities, plaque, and bad breath. Add extra protection by brushing with a fluoride toothpaste that fights both gingivitis and plaque. Crest Gum Care and Colgate Total are two you can try.

Zinc: a zinger for good looks

People with hair loss problems often have low levels of zinc, according to some research. Although there is no evidence that taking zinc will encourage new hair growth, you should try to get enough of this health-promoting mineral. Because zinc is also good for teeth and gums, you may also give your smile a boost. The recommended dietary allowance for men is 11 mg, but adult women only need 8 mg. You can get zinc from meat, pumpkin seeds, dairy products, whole grains, oysters, peanuts or lima beans.

Protein builds strong hair and nails

Brittle hair can mean bad hair days for men and women alike. Protein is vital to building stronger hair, so be sure you get as much as you need. The U.S. government recommends around 4 grams of protein for every 11 pounds of body weight – roughly 36 grams for a 100-pound adult. Get your protein from such foods as lean meats, grains, low-fat dairy foods, nuts, eggs, and beans.

Two protein building blocks – arginine and cysteine – are essential for hair growth. In fact, your hair follicles must have these amino acids to produce strands of hair. Some even think that these amino acids may make your nails stronger, too. Although liquid supplements from a health store may be necessary, start by getting your amino acids from food. You can get ample arginine from peanuts, walnuts, seeds, whole grains, rice, beans, and gelatin. Find cysteine in chickpeas (garbanzo beans), lentils, and from cheeses such as mozzarella, cheddar, and Swiss.

The right recipe for slumber

A National Sleep Foundation survey reports that 63 percent of American adults get less than eight hours of sleep. Live like this and exhaustion may not be your only problem. Some think a lack of sleep raises your adrenalin, which can push your cholesterol levels up – and that's not good for your heart. To keep from tiring out your heart as well as the rest of your body, nibble these nutrients to help you hibernate. You may get more sleep and help your cholesterol take a nosedive, too.

Boost melatonin for restful sleep

Remember the last time you had that urge to drift off to sleep in a nice dark room? That was a sign that the hormone, melatonin, was doing its job. Melatonin is produced in the pineal gland at the base of your brain. More melatonin helps you sleep, while dwindling melatonin triggers alertness in daylight. So how can you boost your melatonin when you're ready to sleep? See red – red from cherries that is. Cherries are chock-full of melatonin. They can help you sleep sounder and wake refreshed.

To raise your chances of sleeping better, experts suggest you eat melatonin-filled foods an hour or two before you go to bed. A handful of cherries would fit the bill quite nicely. In fact, snacking on cherries could be especially important for older adults, because the body produces less melatonin as you age. Other high-melatonin foods include oats, sweet corn, bananas, tomato soup, and rice. Try each and see which one works best for you.

Carb-tryptophan team makes you drowsy

Pair carbohydrates with the amino acid tryptophan, and you'll be on your way to dreamland in no time. In addition to getting melatonin from food, you can give your body the ingredients it needs to make more melatonin on its own.

Tryptophan is one of those special ingredients. Found in protein-rich foods like turkey, dairy products, tuna, pumpkin seeds, and nuts, tryptophan is converted to serotonin, then melatonin, in your brain. Serotonin helps regulate your sleep cycle and is associated with a peaceful, relaxed feeling. In other words, serotonin starts the job that melatonin is designed to finish – helping you drift off to dreamland. But to get this process started, tryptophan needs to get to your brain quickly. That's where carbohydrates come in. To give tryptophan its all-expenses-paid cruise to your brain, eat foods like pasta, grains, corn, potatoes, and beans along with your protein. Try a tasty twosome like tuna on whole wheat or cereal with milk. Combinations like these team up to deliver just what it takes to make you drowsy.

Calcium sends you to dreamland

Calcium is another crucial ingredient in the recipe for melatonin. Milk, with its soothing tryptophan, is a good source of calcium as well, but yogurt, kale, and sardines can help, too. Most adults under 50 need at least 1,000 milligrams (mg) of calcium each day while older adults should get 1,200 mg. What's more, Russel J. Reiter, author of *Melatonin: Your Body's Natural Wonder Drug,* suggests that taking 1,000 mg of calcium with 500 mg of magnesium right before bed may help you sleep better at night. If you're considering using supplements for this strategy, check with your doctor first.

Ease your stress with magnesium

Magnesium is not only needed to make melatonin, it may also ease stress. Yugoslavian researchers found that people under chronic stress had low magnesium levels – which actually made their stress worse. If you're stressed out, it's probably harder to get to sleep. You need to keep your magnesium from dropping off, so you won't have trouble dropping off to sleep. Spread peanut butter on whole grain crackers, or mine more magnesium from nuts and green leafy vegetables.

You may need to talk to your doctor about supplements if you're on a high-protein diet. That's because you're probably eating lots of meat, fish, and dairy products – all foods low in magnesium. Supplements may be necessary to keep you from becoming deficient.

B vitamins end tossing and turning

Keep the right B vitamins around to help you keep the melatonin coming. Your body can use tryptophan to make either niacin (vitamin B3) or melatonin. If you find yourself tossing and turning, try to get extra niacin into your diet, so your body can make melatonin instead of B3 from your tryptophan reserves. Dried apricots, peanuts, barley, chicken, and turkey are good sources of niacin.

Vitamin B6 helps convert tryptophan to serotonin. Older adults are at risk for B6 shortage, but they're not the only ones. You may also lack vitamin B6 if you smoke, drink alcohol, take birth control pills or estrogen, have carpal tunnel syndrome, suffer from depression, or eat a lot of refined foods. To boost your B6, eat avocados, bananas, carrots, rice, and shrimp. To get B3 and B6 together, eat brewer's yeast, salmon, sunflower seeds, tuna, and wheat bran.

Keys to mental fitness 5

Tap into the power of your mind

The fountain of youth isn't an exercise program or a super food –
although both help. It's simply positive thinking. Apparently, the saying
"you're only as old as you feel" is more fact than fiction. Recent studies
suggest having an optimistic view of aging can add seven and a half years
to your life – just one example of how many aspects of aging are all in
your mind.

■ Research into the mind-body connection shows that positive emotions can strengthen your immune system and help you fight disease. When you're sick, your emotions can help you mend, sometimes as much as medicine can.

Often, a strong desire to live is the only explanation when a critically ill person recovers – and survives. A willingness to fight for your health can mean the difference between life and death.

■ Good mental health protects your relationships. These, in turn, can lengthen your life.

■ A positive view of life gives you incentive to keep your body healthy. You're more likely to follow proper nutrition, pursue exercise, and build solid self-esteem.

Improve your health with an improved attitude

Mental fitness is not just staying sharp with crossword puzzles. It's more
about a mindset that expects – and fights for – good health.

Take Rich, for example. In his mid-forties, he found out cancer had spread to his spine. Doctors gave him less than a 5 percent chance of survival. Discouraged, he put his affairs in order, and prayed that God would take care of his wife and 7-year-old daughter when he was gone. "All my initial efforts went towards giving up to what appeared to be the inevitable," he said.

Then one day he had a big change of attitude. "I decided to forget the odds. Whatever this demon was that was supposed to claim me was going to have to fight me to do it. I started looking at myself as living with cancer instead of dying of cancer."

His hope and faith kept him going through grueling treatments. "I also knew being in excellent shape and having good mental training discipline was a great asset – so I put those to work for me." Just six months later, he showed no signs of living cancer cells.

Rich credits his recovery to his positive attitude. "Don't ever give up on yourself," he advises. "Give your body all it needs for the fight. But first, and foremost, you've got to believe in yourself."

With optimism, the love and support of his family, and doctors who believe in him, Rich is winning his battle against cancer. He truly believes attitude is everything.

Opt for optimism

If you're an optimist, you know you have inside whatever it takes to make it through tough times. You don't paste on a happy face and ignore sorrow or trouble. In fact, you probably feel deeply. You simply control the intensity of those feelings – not allowing them to overwhelm you. Perhaps because of this positive attitude, optimists tend to live longer than pessimists.

If looking for that silver lining doesn't come naturally, don't be discouraged. Optimism can be learned. Here are a few tricks to get you started.

- Smile. If you turn on a high-wattage grin – one that raises your cheeks – you'll really feel happier. Research proves your emotions follow your expression, not the other way around.

- Resist negative thoughts. See yourself as a success, and failure will become the exception rather than the rule.

- Put it all in perspective. Ask yourself if this will matter in five years.

- If you catch yourself too often thinking, "I wish I were a…," try finishing this sentence instead: "I'm glad I'm not a…" By comparing yourself to others who are less fortunate, you create a more positive, satisfied view of your life.

Redefine aging

Do you approach your golden years with anticipation? Remember Robert Browning's famous line, "Grow old along with me! The best is yet to be."

Or is your definition of aging closer to that of the English author Anthony Powell who once said, "Growing old is like being increasingly penalized for a crime you haven't committed."

In this century, aging doesn't necessarily mean becoming sick or frail. A recent survey by the National Council on the Aging found that a majority of adults over 65 defined their health as "good" or "excellent" while less than 30 percent considered themselves in "fair to poor" health.

Compared to results from the same survey done 30 years ago, today's seniors feel better, and also have fewer worries about finances, health, crime, and loneliness than their counterparts did in the 70s.

In addition, as people age, they're less likely to experience negative feelings and they generally feel more joy in and appreciation for life. So abandon all your old notions about aging and adopt new, more positive ones.

Elizabeth Arden, famous for her beauty products, once said, "I'm not interested in age. People who tell me their age are silly. You're as old as you feel." Tape that to your mirror, start believing it, and you might be surprised how much better your golden years are.

Take control of your emotions

How you feel about yourself is key to being happy and satisfied with your life. Direct your emotions onto a positive path and the happiness will follow.

Love yourself to live longer

You know the little voice in your head that says you're only as valuable as what you achieve? Learn to ignore it. True self-esteem comes from understanding that you can have value that is independent of any particular achievement. Know this, and you become a stronger, more secure person.

Best of all, feel good about yourself and you'll live longer – and healthier. You are less likely to use drugs, or suffer from ulcers and sleepless nights. You'll generally take better care of your health and feel better about the world. Here's how to boost your self-esteem.

■ Would you let someone spread lies about you? That's what your little voice does. Listen to your internal conversation and you will hear its put-downs. When you catch yourself being critical, respond by saying, "Stop it," or remind yourself of what is false and what is true.

■ Everyone has rules to live by. Take a look at yours. If you're holding yourself up to some impossible standard of perfection, you will always feel like a failure. Write more reasonable rules and take pleasure in doing the best you can.

■ Learn from your mistakes but move on. Set a time limit on how long you punish yourself for past failures. This way, they can't handicap your future.

■ Take the driver's seat, especially in roles you value – be it parent, grandparent, provider, homemaker, or volunteer. People who control the most important role in their lives live longer and are happier. On the other hand, studies show those without a feeling of control in these roles are more likely to smoke, drink, and suffer from obesity – all risk factors for premature death.

■ Indulge a passion that fuels the deepest part of you. Fearlessly pursue a worthy goal and you will find creative ways to overcome any obstacle. Research shows that you will be happiest when investing in something you care about.

Set a new course for happiness

Ever had the hankering to fly a plane or take a cooking class? Now is the time to do all the things you may have put off. Learning new skills keeps your mind fresh and your motivation for life high.

Before you choose a new hobby, however, take these things into account.

■ List your strengths and weaknesses so you don't sell yourself short or overwork your body.

■ Cut intimidating projects into manageable bites. You will gain a sense of accomplishment as you complete each step.

■ Manage your time so your activities match your values and goals. Spend the majority of your time on the things that matter most to you.

■ Throw yourself an appreciation party. After all, you have accomplished much, and you should celebrate the positive instead of moaning about the negative.

■ Some interests are better shared. Check the listings at your community center for classes that will bring you in contact with like-minded people.

Remember, no one can make the same contribution to the world that you can.

___

Fend off hurt feelings

Living under a cloud of hurt feelings is bad for your health. The good news is, you have more control over your feelings than you think. Here's a simple tool, called cognitive therapy, which can help put things in perspective.

■ Divide a page into four columns.

■ In the first, describe a painful event as you remember it. (For example, a friend didn't say hello at the supermarket.)

■ In the next column, write down your first impression or belief about the event. (She ignored me on purpose; nobody likes me.)

■ In the third column, write how this made you feel. (Rejected; hurt) Think a little about your reaction. Did you take it too personally or blow it out of proportion? Can the situation be interpreted in a different light? If you change your first impression, you can often deflect the bad feelings that follow.

- In the fourth column, write down a more positive response to the whole situation. (Perhaps she didn't see me or she had something else on her mind; next time I will say hello first.)

Did any of these words crop up in your second column: should, always, never, everybody, nobody, ought, must, and must have? These can make you feel pressured or resentful, or represent blanket statements that are rarely true. Try to see the event through a stranger's eye, and you can often re-interpret it to lessen your stress and anger.

Learn to forgive

Letting go of anger and resentment is good for your mind and your body. According to research if you forgive:

- you'll suffer less stress and depression, and their unhealthy symptoms.

- you'll have generally fewer health problems.

- you'll feel better psychologically and emotionally.

- you'll increase your self-confidence and enjoy better relationships.

Holding on to this kind of pain doesn't harm the person who wronged you, but your body's response – a rise in blood pressure, anxiety levels, and stress – may increase your risk of heart disease and cancer.

Remember, forgiveness doesn't necessarily mean you reconcile with the person who hurt you, or that you do not pursue justice. It just means you let go of the blame and the pain. This way you regain power over your own emotions.

5 easy stress solutions

You know stress wreaks havoc on your health – in fact it impacts almost every system in your body. It not only increases your risk of a heart attack, it can worsen irritable bowel syndrome, bring on asthma attacks, cause migraines, and even affect your arthritis or psoriasis.

Finding ways to cope with daily stress is essential to staying and feeling young. Many experts believe your brain is possibly your strongest weapon against this aspect of life and aging. Here are some cutting-edge theories from top scientists to help you de-stress.

Let faith bring you peace

There is a growing amount of scientific research that shows people with a strong, active religion are healthier, often live longer, and generally deal better with life's difficulties than those who are nonreligious. Many find believing in a higher power to be an immense source of comfort and peace. These people are usually more optimistic about the future because they believe events are part of a bigger plan. Having what is called a "prayerful, prayerlike" attitude – one of devotion and acceptance – can help you deal with stress.

Quiet your thoughts

Just 20 minutes of focused relaxation a day could lengthen your life, lower your blood pressure and cholesterol, improve your mental health, and reduce chronic pain, anxiety, and stress. Here's how to discover the health benefits for yourself.

- Find a quiet spot and rest comfortably. Take the phone off the hook, if necessary, and make sure you'll have no other distractions.

- Close your eyes, breathe deeply, and relax all your muscles.

- Think of a word or phrase with special meaning to you. It should be something uplifting, like the word "joy," or "peace." Or choose a favorite verse or prayer. Reflect on it quietly, pushing aside intrusive thoughts.

- Continue to relax like this for about 10 to 20 minutes.

Try eating strawberries to reduce stress and calm anxiety. You'll get a surge of dopamine, an ingredient in the brain chemical norepinephrine, which controls how well you deal with stress.

Meditation works best when you focus on someone or something else, ignoring fears and problems.

Be mindful of the moment

When was the last time you noticed the tickle of peach fuzz on your lips, or how socks feel on your feet? Stress crops up when you worry about the future. If you can focus on the moment, the future and its problems will melt away. A practical example of this is called mindfulness, which requires you notice and accept the sensations and thoughts you experience as they happen.

This can be easier than you think. Start by learning how to really pay attention to your breathing.

■ Relax and follow your breath in and out. Notice the beginning, middle, and end of each in-breath.

■ Do the same with each out-breath. Notice the rise and fall of your chest or abdomen. Don't try to breathe any differently from your normal breathing.

■ Continue breathing slowly and evenly – with awareness – for 10 to 20 minutes.

Now practice this same mindfulness during your everyday activities. Chew your food slowly, for example, tasting every bite, and notice the different textures in your mouth. Experts believe mindfulness can bring on positive changes in how your brain and immune system respond to stress and disease.

Loosen tense muscles

Just like ice cream heads straight for the hips, stress tends to get trapped in tight muscles. For example, holding on to stress can cause crippling back and shoulder pain. To release your muscles, try simple progressive relaxation.

■ Find a comfortable position and begin breathing slowly and deeply.

■ Tense the muscles in your toes for a count of 10.

■ Release them slowly and completely while you count to 10.

■ Next tense the muscles of your feet in the same way.

■ Continue up the entire length of your body, tensing and relaxing every muscle group.

■ By the time you reach the top of your head, you should feel completely relaxed.

Let laughter into your life

The cheapest medicine around – a bout of good humor – can put pain and problems in perspective. Studies show laughter lowers stress levels and boosts your immune system.

- Laughter can relieve pain. But humor works best this way if you choose your own "medicine." So pick out your favorite comedy the next time you visit the video store and laugh your pain away.

- Joke fall flat? Laugh anyway. Even forced laughter will improve your mood.

The average child laughs about 300 times a day, but most adults only 17 times. Add some silliness to your life and find your inner child.

- Check the TV listings for good comedies a week in advance. Anticipating mirth boosts your immune system about as much as the actual laughing does.

Bring others on the journey

Loved ones touch your heart in many ways. Amazing research about relationships and longevity shows a large support group lowers stress levels, blood pressure, and your risk of heart disease and heart attacks. Face it, having friends and family around can mean a healthier, longer life.

- **Keep a partner.** If you're happily married, odds are you'll live longer and have fewer medical problems than your single, widowed, or divorced counterparts. Not only are spouses a great source of support and social fun, but your life partner tends to watch out for your health, insuring that both of you get the best medical care. Men, especially, seem to benefit from being married.

- **Reach out to others.** Variety may not only be the spice of life, it seems to mean a longer life, too! Take this advice to heart and widen your circle to include those outside your normal social group. Nurture friendships with teens and young adults. Their youth and enthusiasm will keep you young, just as your wisdom can help them grow. Consider volunteering or mentoring if you find yourself isolated from new people. Whether it's church or a weekly card game, being involved in a community keeps you connected and optimistic. Socializing this way is also associated with fewer deaths from all causes combined.

■ **Make a furry friend.** A dog is man's best friend for a reason. The unconditional love from a pet, and the physical touch you lavish on it can both reduce stress. But you don't have to stick with just dogs. Even a goldfish can calm you down and improve your mood.

Best blues-busting secrets

Feeling down? Sadness is just one of the many moods that make up your colorful emotional palate. But if your life looks more like a Rembrandt than a Monet, try these easy tips to turn sadness into joy.

■ **Stop and smell the flowers.** Pleasant scents like lavender, citrus, frankincense, and cedar can lift a dark mood. Experiment with essential oils used for aromatherapy, but follow directions carefully.

■ **Exercise.** Your brain releases feel-good chemicals when you work your muscles.

■ **Tap into touch.** Massage is often as emotionally satisfying as it is physically relaxing.

■ **Catch some sun.** Too little light in your days can really drag you down. Sit outside, turn on some lamps, and raise the shades to lift your mood.

■ **Spill the beans.** Tell a close friend or write in a journal. It will help you process your sadness and move on.

Feeling blue is not the same as being depressed. Clinical depression is a serious condition and needs to be professionally treated. Make sure you see your doctor if your weight changes dramatically, your sleep patterns change, you have mood swings, or you consider suicide. Depression is more common than ever, but there are effective cures. Just as your mind can help heal your body, modern medicine can help heal your mind.

Exercise: the secret to staying young

6

Get moving to live longer and feel younger

A little motion could be your anti-aging potion. Study after study suggests that keeping physically active may help people live longer. In fact, just a bit of exercise might make you feel as if you've turned back the clock.

Add life to your years

How can one 70-year-old be energetic and strong while another can barely walk? Revolutionary new research offers a startling answer. Many abilities we think we lose because of aging we actually lose because of a simple lack of activity. Our bodies may be wasting away from lack of use – not old age.

When it comes to agility and physical power, think of it as a use-it-or-lose-it deal. Start working even a few muscles and you may be astonished at how much power you can keep.

Although Anne is nearly 80 years old, she uses exercise to keep going in spite of joint problems. "With a bad hip and a bad knee," she says, "you've just got to keep moving. Otherwise, they can freeze up on you. A lot of us – at 80 – are playing tennis. It's a game that you can keep on playing so long as you play doubles. Doubles is the answer to anybody our age."

Almost any activity can help you hang on to more of the physical abilities you've got. It might even help restore some of the stamina, flexibility, and muscle tone that have slipped away.

"You've got to be an 'I can' person instead of an 'I can't' person," says Anne. "You have to push yourself and you have to have the right attitude. I don't know what else you do." Major scientific publications seem to agree with Anne.

- Starting at age 40, inactive people lose 8 percent of their lung function every 10 years. But one study suggests that regular exercise can improve your ability to use oxygen so much that it's almost like reversing 20 years of aging.

- Another research team studied over 7,000 people aged 60 to 94. According to their results, inactive seniors could prevent up to half the physical decline blamed on aging. How? Simply by finding fun or convenient ways to make moderate exercise a regular part of life.

- Although most people lose about 15 percent of their muscle between 30 and 80, lifting weights can help – even if the weights are small. Several studies find that strength training can bring back significant muscle power – fairly quickly.

  And that's not all. When it comes to muscle tone and heart health, older men can benefit from strength training as much as younger men. Experts even say that a fit 70-year-old can be as strong as an inactive, unfit 30-year-old.

- You can thrive at 95. According to researchers, people as old as 96 may be able to increase muscle strength and size by up to 200 percent – and they can do it in just eight weeks. Even a little extra muscle power can make a big difference in what you're able to do every day.

The people in these studies aren't Olympic athletes or national champions. They're just normal folks who decided to see what benefits exercise might hold for them. Imagine what could happen when you try it.

Add years to your life

Could keeping too still make you ill? Authorities say that couch potatoes have a higher risk of diseases ranging from arthritis to cancer and beyond. According to some estimates, inactivity causes the deaths of 250,000 people a year in the United States alone. Experts call this threat Sedentary Death Syndrome (SeDS).

You won't need a shot or a pill to prevent SeDS – just look for ways to get more active. Even small amounts of activity may help as long as you keep at it.

What's more, you don't have to be a spring chicken to benefit. Even if you don't start exercising until you're in your 60s, you can still cut your risk of death and disease. A new study by the Centers for Disease Control and Prevention suggests that inactive women over 65 can make surprising gains if they get more active. They could cut their risk of dying from cancer in half and from heart disease by up to 36 percent. Naturally, people who are the most active reap the most life-extending benefits, but even moderate exercise may help you live longer.

So, get a notion to get in motion and start looking and feeling younger than your years. One thing's for sure, stretching your legs may stretch your lifespan.

---

5 easy ways to get more active

■ Take a walk through a local park or garden.

■ Go bowling with friends or family.

■ Lift hand-held weights as you talk on the phone.

■ Rock in a rocking chair.

■ Dance as you perform household chores.

Reap big rewards with a little exercise

Like an unexpected care package, exercise can be full of pleasant surprises. Physical activity is packed with perks that can make you happier and healthier. In fact, the list of benefits is so long that it's impossible to include everything, but here are a few examples.

Fight fatigue

You might think you don't have the energy to exercise now that you're older, but exercise will actually give you a natural energy boost. Even a 10-minute workout may foil fatigue – because it releases chemicals in your brain that improve your mood. In addition, make physical activity a regular part of your day, and you could soon feel as peppy as a 25-year-old.

At 50, Marcy has discovered that just daily stretches and frequent walking can make a difference. "I stretch no more than 10 minutes every morning, and I do whatever I can to get my walking in – anything. I used to try to avoid stairs and now I go up as many as I can. I feel much more energetic now," she declares.

Can people with a disability or chronic condition get active?

Researchers have found that regular physical activity can improve your health even if you are frail, disabled, or coping with disease – particularly if you stick with it long-term.

Don't be discouraged if you have a chronic condition, like asthma, or congestive heart failure. You may still be able to exercise during those times when your condition is under control. Programs even exist for the bed-ridden and those unable to stand.

Before you begin, talk to your doctor about your condition and the types of exercise it's safe for you to do.

And if that natural energy boost from getting active isn't enough, exercise also improves your ability to fall asleep and sleep well. So if lack of sleep is the reason your get-up-and-go has got up and went, a little physical activity could have you feeling more peppy soon.

Fire up your immunity

Keep your immune system humming at full power and you're less likely to get sick.

Regular moderate exercise can make sure your immune system stays charged up by stimulating white blood cells called macrophages.

These "natural killer cells" circulate throughout your body fighting invaders, like viruses and bacteria.

And the older you are, the more you may benefit from being in good physical shape. For example, according to research, women over 67 who walk or exercise regularly have fewer respiratory infections than others. It's almost as if illness has a tougher time hitting a moving target. So catch up with some exercise and you just might avoid catching whatever's "going around."

Look like a million

Marcy believes her exercise routine has helped her look and feel better. "I know I've lost inches because of it. And my husband has even mentioned that I look good."

As you get more active, you'll build stronger muscles that can help protect your spinal column and improve your posture. A better posture can add polish to – and take years off – your appearance.

You can also get a leg up on looking good by dodging varicose veins. Walking, swimming, and yoga can give your leg muscles the good workout they need to resist those unsightly lines. On top of that, you may also end up with legs that are more toned, attractive, and eye-catching. If you already suffer from varicose veins, just don't overdo it.

Exercise saves you money. According to a survey, active Americans over the age of 15 saved an annual average of $330 in medical costs compared to folks who were inactive.

Best of all, many types of exercise can lead to better muscle tone – and not just in your legs. Frank Garver, a 50-year-old who swims and lifts weights regularly says, "I can tell I've traded fat for muscle in my arms and shoulders and, to a lesser extent, in my neck and back. My shirts are tighter through the shoulders and only my newer ones fit."

John is 65 and originally took up running to see if it would help him lose weight. "Not only did running prove to be an exquisite solution to my weight problem – the pounds fell off – but I could eat just about anything I wanted." He doesn't believe running necessarily ensures a long life, but says, "It just makes the life one has that much more enjoyable."

Recharge a sluggish metabolism

As you grow older, your metabolism slows down and you burn fewer calories. If you still eat the same number of calories every day – but burn fewer of them – you can't help but gain weight. If only you could find a way to speed that metabolism back up.

Simple strength exercises can help. Whether you call it strength training, resistance training, or weight training, you're building muscle by lifting some type of weight. But the best news is that it may revitalize your metabolism, help you lose weight, and make you stronger. It's a three-for-one deal that could literally lighten your load.

You'll learn just how easy and beneficial strength training can be when you read the *Power up to slim down* chapter.

Give your digestive system a tune-up

If you're plagued by poor digestion, the answer may be at your feet. A daily brisk walk – or any other moderate exercise – can ease constipation enough that you can throw away those pills and powders. This "natural laxative" can help your digestive system work smoothly – without any of the unpleasant side effects that come from harsh laxatives.

That daily walk may also be enough to cut your ulcer risk in half, according to one study. While moderate, regular exercise can benefit anyone, men, especially, were protected against ulcers in the upper intestine. Try walking or jogging at least a mile and a half every day."

Move with ease

Becoming more active could also be your ticket to better balance, greater flexibility, and, perhaps, added strength. You need all three of these to reach, bend, stoop, and climb stairs easily. What's more, balance, strength, and flexibility also help prevent the falls that can lead to disabling injuries. The flowing, dance-like moves of tai chi are one way to achieve these goals. You can learn more about this in *3 paths to better balance*.

Dodge deadly diseases

Heart disease, stroke, cancer, and diabetes are dangerous, devastating conditions. Yet physical activity can help fight them all.

For instance, walk 30 to 45 minutes three times a week and cut your heart attack risk in half. Here's what else exercise can do for heart health.

■ Reduce the risk of a second heart attack.

■ Cut triglycerides and total cholesterol.

■ Lower the risk of developing high blood pressure.

- Keep resting blood pressure rates lower for hours after an exercise session ends.

- Shrink your chances of developing and dying from heart disease.

Frank feels good about how his swimming and strength-training regimen may have helped his heart. "As part of a wellness physical about a year ago, I had a baseline EKG," he says. "The cardiologist said my heart was in excellent shape and that I have less than a 5 percent chance of a heart attack."

Physical activity can help fight other deadly or disabling diseases too.

- Keeping active may lower your risk of cancer, especially colon and breast cancer.

- Moderate exercise – such as walking an hour a day – may slash your risk of type 2 diabetes in half. What's more, this type of activity also lowers blood glucose, pushing it closer to normal. So, if you enjoy a brisk walk or do other moderate activities for fun, these hobbies can help you fight diabetes. Just remember, if you already have diabetes, check with your doctor before starting any exercise program.

- Make physical activity your ally against the brittle bones of osteoporosis and its dangers. Weight-bearing exercises, such as gardening or lifting weights, can help you keep and build strong bones. Ask your doctor about exercises that will strengthen large leg muscles to help prevent falls and fractures. Even if you already have osteoporosis, walking, jogging, lifting light weights, gardening, and dancing may help.

- If you suffer from arthritis, exercise can increase your strength and flexibility and reduce the amount of medication needed to control pain. It may even delay or prevent arthritis from developing in other joints. Walk, swim, and cycle to help increase your mobility and decrease joint pain and stiffness.

Doctors often recommend movement to decrease low back pain. Ask your doctor for specific exercises that can help.

- Yale University researchers discovered that men who walked over a mile a day cut their risk of stroke in half.

- Ease the symptoms of fibromyalgia with low-impact aerobics like swimming or riding a stationary bike. These activities get your heart pumping and boost the oxygen needed to fuel your muscles. You may feel pain and discomfort at first, so start slowly and build up to working out several times each week.

Boost your brainpower

Aerobic exercise feeds your brain cells with oxygen and nutrients. That may be why physical activity can encourage creativity and speed your thinking. Exercise can also tighten up your reaction time and help you process information faster.

With your brain working at full capacity, you've got a better chance of solving problems clearly and making well-reasoned decisions. Fascinating new research finds that physical activity may ward off Alzheimer's, one of the most dreaded senior diseases. Exercise increases brain chemicals that help the growth of new brain nerve cells.

Dr. Susan Spalding, a Certified Movement Analyst, is Director of Dance Programs at Berea College in Kentucky. She explains why dancing – such as square dancing or contra dancing – might give you a leg up on brainpower. "It helps memory, because of the complex coordinations involved. It helps with both short-term and long-term memory, and has been recommended as a defense against Alzheimer's disease," she says.

A study out of Case Western Reserve University School of Medicine in Ohio supports the theory that regular exercise – especially between the ages of 20 and 60 – may lower your chances of getting Alzheimer's disease. Experts emphasize that the exercise must be done over the long-term to have any effect.

The bottom line: to stay sage as you age, get active. Running, swimming, tennis, weight training, biking, and golf are examples of exercise that will do your brain – and your body – good.

Easy steps to a fit future

Anyone can exercise. It can even be convenient, cheap, and fun! Forget about the young, athletic bodies you've seen in gym TV ads. You don't have to fit into that mold. Make exercise fit you instead.

You can learn innovative exercises to use in your own home that are so easy your friends will think you've been working out every day at the gym. On the other hand, you may want to take a class or use exercise machines at a fitness center.

If you like organized exercise, learn from a trainer or class instructor to be sure you know how to do the exercise correctly. You'll get better results and suffer fewer injuries. With just a little information and a few preparations, you can find the perfect fitness activities for you.

Screen trainers or exercise class instructors by asking if they are certified to work with older adults.

John discovered how easy fitness could be when he took up running to lose weight. "I never had any real athletic ability, but this was something I could do – at my own pace and convenience – and requiring minimal investment," he says. "I still enjoy it immensely more than 40 years later."

Although running works for John, you're free to choose anything you like – as long as it works well for you. In fact, you could already be physically active and not even know it. If you spent 10 minutes planting flowers in your yard this morning, another 10 briskly walking around the block after lunch, and 10 more minutes raking leaves, you've put in a good 30-minute workout.

Even sex and dancing count as healthy exercise. Both burn calories and give your muscles a workout, so either one can contribute to better health and fitness.

On top of that, routine tasks such as cleaning the house can increase your fitness level. At 66, Ann Akers is a record-setting marathon runner. Yet when she started her housecleaning business, she discovered that simple cleaning tasks – like vacuuming under a bed – worked different muscles and improved her fitness.

One thing's for sure, you don't have to be miserable while you get fit. You don't even have to go to a gym, lift heavy weights, or do hours of strenuous exercise. You can look forward to health benefits even if you only rack up 30 minutes of moderate activity each day.

Fighting cancer with fitness

Rich Horning has run marathons before, but now he faces a larger – and deadlier – challenge. The 46-year-old was diagnosed with esophageal cancer that later spread to his spine. Given less than a 5 percent chance to survive, he decided to fight.

"I wasn't going to let it ruin my life," he declares. "I took a new pair of running shoes off my closet shelf and renewed my subscription to *Runner's World*. I was now training for the race of my life."

That race soon included monthly chemotherapy treatments. Between sessions, he continued to run four to five times each week, lift weights two to three times a week, and play golf and tennis.

"It's all with a different goal and attitude now though," he explains. "I seldom run hard or lift heavy. It's all for maintaining the best fitness level I can to help my body stay as healthy as possible to fight the disease."

Rich works closely with his doctors and is careful not to overtax his body. He takes a nap after running, eats well, drinks plenty of water, and works hard to stay positive. His doctors are impressed. "During my checkups, they were amazed at my continued good appearance, attitude, and lack of problems," Rich comments. "They said whatever I was doing, to just keep doing it."

After six months of chemotherapy, Rich learned he beat the odds and was cancer-free. He believes exercise helped him win his battle. "No matter what your fitness condition is now, you need some fitness, rest, and good nutrition for the fight," he advises. "Chemo drugs are toxic and tough on the heart and blood. Help get them both back in shape between chemo sessions to give your body a fighting chance."

Add activity throughout your day

If you're just starting to become more active, try taking your exercise in "bite-size" portions.

Plan three 10-minute sessions throughout the day. Soon, you'll be able to do 30 minutes of moderate activity all at once. If you're wondering what counts as moderate exercise, try the "talk test."

For winning results, experts suggest you aim for 30 minutes of exercise at least three days out of the week. If you can step up to four days or more, that's even better.

Any activity that causes you to breathe hard but still lets you talk – without gasping for breath – counts as moderate exercise for you. This is called the talk test.

Get expert advice

Your doctor can be your greatest champion in your quest for fitness. In fact, before you begin any exercise, talk with her about the best activities for you. Here are a few good questions to ask.

- Is it safe for me to do the exercises that I have planned?

- How can I find out whether I'm exercising hard enough? How can I keep from exercising too hard?

- Are there any sports or exercises I should avoid?

- Do I have any health conditions – or do I take any medications – that could affect my exercise plans?

- Are there any exercises or activities that would be particularly helpful to me?

Stick with activities that can give you the most fun and health benefits and the least chance of trouble.

Find your fitness level

Finding out how fit you are – or even how fit you aren't – helps you tailor a fitness plan to your needs. After all, no adult is typical. So, don't worry if you're not a tough-as-nails athlete. Simply become more active and you'll start feeling the benefits and seeing the results. To determine your fitness, try the one-mile fitness test.

The one-mile fitness test

This is a way to get a rough measure of your fitness. First you'll need a one-mile course on a safe, flat surface. Either use a measured track at a nearby school or park — most tracks are one-quarter mile so you'll need to do four laps — or mark a route you're comfortable with. Always perform the test on the same course so you can compare results.

Use a watch with a second hand to time yourself, and see how long it takes to walk the course. Walk as fast as you can, keeping a constant pace and breathing evenly.

At the end of the course, record how long — in minutes and seconds — it took you to walk the mile. You'll probably be somewhere between 10 and 20 minutes.

Now keep walking slowly and take your pulse. Locate a pressure point at your wrist, temple, or throat where you can feel your artery throbbing. Gently touch the point and count how many times your heart beats during a 6-second time period. Multiply that by 10 — or just add a zero to your number — and you have your heartbeats per minute.

Now find your age range on the following chart, and go to the row with your heart rate. Round up or down if you have to. Make sure you're checking under the appropriate sex column and find your time for the one-mile walk. You can see your approximate fitness level — high, average, or low.

One-mile fitness test

Age	Heart rate	Men: fitness level			Women: fitness level		
		High less than	**Average** between	**Low** more than	**High** less than	**Average** between	**Low** more than
40s	110	15:38	15:38-18:05	18:05	17:20	17:20-19:15	19:15
	120	15:09	15:09-17:36	17:36	16:50	16:50-18:45	18:45
	130	14:41	14:41-17:07	17:07	16:24	16:24-18:18	18:18
	140	14:12	14:12-16:38	16:38	15:54	15:54-17:48	17:48
	150	13:42	13:42-16:09	16:09	15:24	15:24-17:18	17:18
	160	13:15	13:15-15:42	15:42	14:54	14:54-16:48	16:48
	170	12:45	12:45-15:12	15:12	14:25	14:25-16:18	16:18
50s	110	15:22	15:22-17:49	17:49	17:04	17:04-18:40	18:40
	120	14:53	14:53-17:20	17:20	16:36	16:36-18:12	18:12
	130	14:24	14:24-16:51	16:51	16:06	16:04-17:42	17:42
	140	13:51	13:51-16:22	16:22	15:36	15:36-17:18	17:18
	150	13:26	13:26-15:53	15:53	15:06	15:06-16:48	16:48
	160	12:59	12:59-15:26	15:26	14:36	14:36-16:18	16:18
	170	12:30	12:30-14:56	14:56	14:06	14:06-15:48	15:48
60+	110	15:33	15:33-17:55	17:55	16:36	16:36-18:00	18:00
	120	15:04	15:04-17:24	17:24	16:06	16:06-17:30	17:30
	130	14:36	14:36-16:57	16:57	15:37	15:37-17:01	17:01
	140	14:07	14:07-16:28	16:28	15:09	15:09-16:31	16:31
	150	13:39	13:39-15:59	15:59	14:39	14:39-16:02	16:02
	160	13:10	13:10-15:30	15:30	14:12	14:12-15:32	15:32
	170	12:42	12:42-15:04	15:04	13:42	13:42-15:04	15:04

3-way fitness test

If weather or physical problems keep you from taking the one-mile fitness test, there are other ways to test your fitness. Just check with your doctor first if you have high blood pressure, dizziness, chest pain, or congestive heart failure. Recruit a partner and stretch and warm up a bit before you start. Do your best but don't push yourself too hard.

30-second chair stand — measures lower body strength

- Sit in a chair without arms that's about 17 inches high. Put your feet flat on the floor. Cross your arms over your chest.

- Count the number of times you can come to a full stand in a 30-second time period.

2-minute step-in-place — measures endurance

- You or your partner find the point midway between your hip and knee. Mark this target height on a table leg or a wall.

- March in place for two minutes and count how often your right knee reaches your target height.

Chair sit-and-reach — measures flexibility

- Brace a straight-back chair, approximately 17 inches high, against a wall and sit on its edge.

- Place one foot flat on the floor and extend the other leg out in front of you with your heel on the floor and your foot flexed.

- Bend forward from your hips, keeping your back straight. Stretch your arms out and try to touch the toes on your extended leg.

- Have your partner measure how many inches are between your fingers and your toes. This will be a negative (-) number if you can't quite reach your toes and a positive (+) number if you can reach beyond your toes.

Adapted, by permission, from R.E.Rikli & C.J.Jones, 1999, "Development and validation of a functional fitness test for community-residing older adults," Journal of Aging and Physical Activity, 7(2):129-161

3-way fitness test average fitness scores

Age	# Stands		# Steps		Reach (in inches)	
	Men	Women	Men	Women	Men	Women
60-64	14-19	13-17	91-112	79-103	-2 to +3	0 to +4
65-69	13-17	12-15	90-113	77-103	-2.5 to +2.5	+0.5 to +4
70-74	12-17	11-15	84-107	72-97	-3 to +2	-0.5 to +3
75-79	12-16	11-14	78-105	72-96	-3.5 to +1	-1 to +3
80-84	10-14	9-13	75-99	64-87	-4.5 to +0.5	-1.5 to +2.5
85-89	9-13	8-12	63-87	59-81	-4.5 to -0.5	-2 to +2

Adapted, by permission, from R.E.Rikli & C.J.Jones, 1999, "Functional fitness normative scores for community-residing older adults, ages 60-94," Journal of Aging and Physical Activity, 7(2):169

Maximize long-term results with target heart rate

Many people use something called a "target heart rate" to make sure they exercise hard enough. Yet some medications and conditions affect your heart rate (HR) and therefore interfere with this type of measurement.

If you'd like to track your fitness efforts using your target heart rate, get your doctor's approval first. Or talk to him about other methods to monitor how hard you exercise.

According to the American Heart Association, your target heart rate range should fall between 50 percent and 75 percent of your maximum heart rate. For top-notch results, maintain your target heart rate for at least 20 minutes.

If your doctor approves, start exercising at 50 percent of your maximum heart rate. Over several weeks, gradually increase how hard you exercise until you reach 75 percent of your maximum heart rate. For example, if you're 55, you'd start near a target heart rate of 83 beats per minute and eventually work up to around 123.

Age	50% of max HR (beats per minute)	75% of max HR (beats per minute)	Maximum HR
40	90	135	180
45	88	131	175
50	85	127	170
55	83	123	165
60	80	120	160
65	78	116	155
70	75	113	150

If you're at a low fitness level, you may need to work below even 50 percent of your target heart rate at first. You can gradually work up to the 50 percent level, then move on to higher levels in your range.

You should never reach your maximum heart rate. In fact, do not try to push yourself up beyond 75 percent without checking with your doctor. If you're not already very physically fit, levels above 75 percent could be dangerous. Call your doctor if you have the following symptoms; you may be in danger from exercising too vigorously.

■ dizziness

■ difficulty breathing

■ nausea

■ pain in your chest, back, left shoulder or arm

If you experience joint pain, extreme fatigue, or problems sleeping, check with your doctor.

Top tips to keep your 'get-up-and-go' going

Whether you're just starting to get fit or you're remodeling your fitness plan, use these tips to help you stay motivated.

- Pick out fitness activities that won't strain your budget.

- Choose activities that you enjoy. After all, why shouldn't fitness be fun?

- Try new sports, games, or exercises from time to time, so you won't get bored. Perhaps schedule aerobic exercises for Mondays, Wednesdays, and Fridays while reserving Tuesdays and Thursdays for strength training.

- Choose activities that fit easily into your daily schedule.

- Make exercise easy and hassle-free. If traffic or weather frequently block you from getting to a gym, you probably won't exercise much. Likewise, if your favorite exercise machine is buried in the back corner of a closet, you probably won't use it.

- Plan for a regular exercise time and block it off on your calendar. Be sure to include time for warming up and cooling down.

- Try to wait at least two hours after a meal before you exercise. Not only will you bypass cramps and other unpleasant effects, you'll also enjoy exercise more when you don't feel full.

- Have a back-up plan. For example, keep an exercise video handy for those days when weather, travel, or even houseguests prevent your usual outdoor exercise or trip to the gym.

- Don't do too much too quickly. If you start slowly, you're not as likely to be discouraged by achy muscles, injuries, or other problems. You can always add more vigorous and interesting exercises later.

Weather tip: Dress in layers so you can add or remove clothes as you feel hotter or colder. Also, drink plenty of water, especially in hot weather.

- Remember to warm up and cool down. Warming up slowly helps protect your heart and muscles. The best way is to just gradually begin whatever activity you'll be doing.

Cooling down helps remove chemical byproducts of exercise from your muscles and bloodstream. To cool down, bring the pace of your workout down slowly. Finish by doing some stretches to help prevent stiffness.

- Avoid overdoing it. Remember that moderate activity gives you health benefits, too. You should feel challenged, but not at your physical limit.

- Get extra incentive from friends and family. Tell them when you reach a goal or have other successes.

- Find an exercise buddy – or even a group or club. Having someone to exercise with can encourage you and keep you from giving up or getting bored.

- Listen to recorded books or music while you work out. Check your local library for tapes or CDs you might enjoy.

- Write down your scores, heart rate, weights and repetitions, or times and notice how they improve. Tracking your progress can make all your efforts worthwhile.

Ann Akers knows the feeling. "You say I have accomplished this, now I'm ready to go to the next step," she explains. "I think it actually improves the health of your body and your mind. You just feel good from accomplishing something."

- If you stop improving, that might be your signal to move up to more challenging activities. Setting a goal can provide incentive.

Learn the terms

If you take a class, watch a video, or use a trainer, you may need to know the terms for the muscle groups you're working. Here's a quick guide.

- **Pectorals, deltoids, and triceps.** Watch someone lying on a weight bench lift a barbell above his chest. This is called a chest or bench press.

  This exercise works the pectoralis major or pecs (your chest muscles), anterior deltoids (front of your shoulders), and triceps (back of your upper arms).

- **Abdominals and obliques.** Listen to almost any ad for a gym and you'll probably hear the word "crunches." Crunches are a little like sit-ups, except you never sit all the way up. Instead, you lift your head and shoulders just far enough to work the stomach muscles. The technique can be tricky, so it's best to learn from an experienced instructor.

Crunches can work lower abdominals or lower abs (your lower stomach), upper abdominals or upper abs (your upper stomach), and external obliques (your sides).

■ **Trapezius and deltoids.** Another common sight in the gym is someone reaching up to pull down a handlebar on a weight machine.

This "pull-down" can strengthen your upper back, including the trapezius or traps (your neck to shoulder) and the posterior deltoids (the back of your shoulders). Some rowing exercises also act on these muscles.

■ **Quadriceps and hamstrings.** Squats and lunges are exercises that build the muscles in and around your upper legs. A squat is a little like trying to sit down on an imaginary chair while a lunge looks like you're trying to go down on one knee.

Exercises like these work the muscles in your gluteus maximus (buttocks), the quadriceps femoris or quads (the front part of your upper legs), and the hamstrings (back of your upper legs).

Check out the muscle diagrams on the following pages. They will help you visualize which muscle group(s) you'll be working during different exercises.

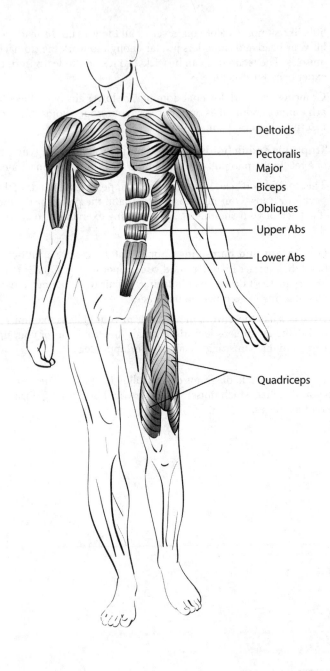

Deltoids

Pectoralis
Major

Biceps

Obliques

Upper Abs

Lower Abs

Quadriceps

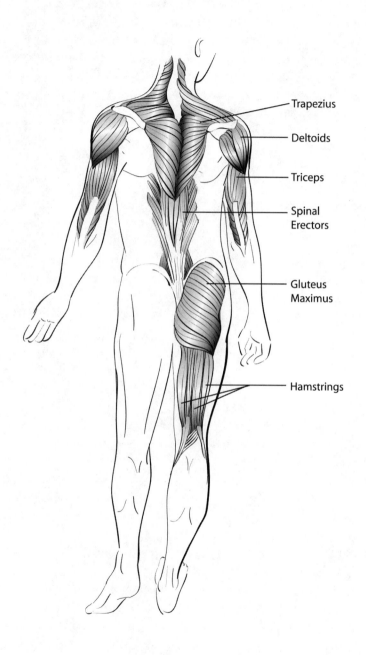

Trapezius

Deltoids

Triceps

Spinal
Erectors

Gluteus
Maximus

Hamstrings

Superstar stretches

7

'Stretch' the benefits of exercise

You can get the fastest fitness improvements from stretching – faster than any other exercise. Still, stretching is the Rodney Dangerfield of the exercise world. It gets no respect. For instance, you may believe stretching is only a chore you're supposed to do before you play a sport. Or worse, you may not stretch at all because you think it's not important.

That's a shame for your body. Stretching is a crucial part of fitness. It helps you get the most from walking, strength training, golf, or whatever other activities you enjoy. On top of that, it's worth doing for its own sake. The more flexible you are, the easier and more pleasant your everyday activities will be.

If you're a beginner, you'll find many easy stretching exercises to start off with. You can choose more challenging stretches if you're already in good shape. No matter which category you fall into, you need to make stretching a key part of your fitness routine.

Loosen up to feel young again

It's natural to get less flexible as you age, but stretching is a natural way to slow and even reverse this process. When you include it in your exercise regimen, you'll quickly notice the improvements. You may become flexible enough to sit on the floor and play with your grandkids. Or you may be able to reach for groceries high up on the supermarket shelf without any help. Here are some of the things stretching can do for you:

■ Stretching will return your muscles to their full range of motion. That may lead to balance and coordination you haven't had for decades, which could reduce your danger of sudden falls or slips. Flexible, fit muscles also mean better posture and fewer everyday aches and pains.

- Your blood may flow better if you stretch. More nutrients will reach your muscles, while waste products will get flushed away.

- A stretched muscle may be at less risk for injury. Or, if your muscle is already injured, stretching could help reduce healing time.

- Stretching is like giving yourself a massage. It helps loosen those knots left behind by the daily grind.

Whether you're young or young at heart, active or wishing you were, stretching is a great way to get in shape. And it may be extra beneficial if you suffer from certain conditions.

Clamp down on muscle cramps

The experts at the American Academy of Orthopaedic Surgeons say tight muscles may have a lot to do with cramps. Stretching seems to get at the root of cramp problems, they suggest, because it lengthens and loosens muscle fibers. These are exciting findings for seniors, since cramps are a major pain in the neck – or leg – for many.

Morning stiffness got you stuck under the covers? Stay in bed and do some of the simple stretches in this chapter to get your morning off to a great start.

During a bout of calf cramps, try stretching the tight muscle by straightening your leg and bending your foot back toward your shin. Hold on to the ball of your foot if necessary. Or if you can stand, put your weight on the aching leg and bend your knee a little. Massaging a cramped muscle can help, too.

To prevent future charley horses, side stitches, and other muscle spasms, make stretching a regular part of your exercise program.

It's also important to drink enough liquids throughout the day. Dehydration is tops on the list of possible cramp causes. If you're active, take in at least six to eight glasses of water a day.

However, cramping may have more serious causes. If stretching and refueling on fluids don't do the trick, let your doctor take a look.

Outwit osteoarthritis

Stretching may seem like the last thing you want to do if you have osteoarthritis. But it may be just what your stiff, painful joints need. It's also what experts prescribe. They suggest stretching every day, or at least every other day. Otherwise, your joints may become stiffer, leaving you with less range of motion. In the long run, you could lose your personal independence when you can't even do your daily chores. By keeping your muscles and tissues strong, they can provide better support and protection for your joints.

If joint pain and swelling seem too daunting, use these tricks of the trade to get relief so you can stretch.

- Apply a heat pack or a steamy towel for 15 to 20 minutes before stretching to help relax your muscles and joints.

- Warm up your muscles with 10 to 15 minutes of light activity like walking. Then follow the stretching instructions later in this chapter.

- Use a cold compress, a bag of ice, or a sack of frozen vegetables after stretching. Apply it for 10 to 15 minutes to reduce joint swelling.

Stretching should be only one part of your exercise routine if you have osteoarthritis. Round out your fitness schedule with strength training and cardio exercises. Always check with your doctor, though, before beginning any of these programs.

Save your bones from a snap

It is especially important to consult with your doctor if you have osteoporosis. This condition leaves your bones brittle and easy to injure. Certain stretches may actually hurt rather than help you. For example, twisting your spine or bending your waist, which you're likely to do while stretching, could break a bone.

You may not even know you have fragile bones. So always ask your doctor if it's safe for you to begin a stretching and exercise routine. If she suspects you're at risk for osteoporosis or any other serious condition, she can give you the necessary tests to know for sure.

Avoid injuries with proper technique

Stretching isn't complicated. Then again, it isn't as simple as leaning one way and reaching another. If you do a stretching maneuver wrong, you won't get all of its benefits or, worse, you could injure yourself. So learn the right way to lean and reach.

Is stretching really necessary?

Stretching may not prevent injury or soreness when you do it before or after an exercise or sport, say scientists in Australia. In fact, they claim stretching may stop an injury only once every 23 years. They came to this startling conclusion after comparing five different stretching studies.

Still, these results are far from proof positive. The study only looked at young healthy adults, so stretching may benefit other groups, such as the elderly. And stretching often gives you a psychological boost. So if it makes you feel better, keep it up. Stretching may or may not prevent soreness and injury, but it will always be a great way to improve your flexibility and increase your range of motion.

Start by knowing when to do it. Remember – stretching is a form of exercise all to itself. So for its own sake, devote at least three times a week to only stretching. If you have a particularly tense or tight part of the body, stretch it every day or even twice a day.

On top of that, stretch along with your daily walk, your tennis match, or your dancing session. Stretching complements every fitness activity under the sun. It's especially important if you're active in physical activities like strength training or cardio. These exercises naturally tighten up your muscles. Stretching counters that by lengthening them.

Whatever activity you're involved in, loosen up lightly before you do it. Then stretch thoroughly afterward. You can skip the first stretch if you're short on time, but make sure to do the end session – before your muscles cool down and tighten up.

Take the crucial first step — warm up

You wouldn't jump into the shower right after turning on the water. The cold water would shock your system. Instead, you'd wait for the water to warm up. It's the same with stretching. Don't dive right in when your muscles are still cold. Spend several minutes warming them up with one of these activities:

- jumping jacks
- a ride on a real or stationary bike
- walking while pumping your arms
- running in place
- practicing the stretches you plan to do
- your favorite exercise or activity at a slow pace

Any one of these can get your heart rate up, loosen your muscles and joints, and prepare you for an injury-free workout.

Work slowly and gently for maximum gain

It's best to stretch all your major muscle groups any time you do a stretching routine. In other words, loosen all the muscles you usually use in your day – your legs, back, neck, and other upper body muscles.

If you're in a rush, however, loosen only the muscles you need at the moment. Work on your legs before you jog, for instance, or stretch your shoulders before golfing. Afterwards, make sure to do a complete stretch. For all your muscles, follow these easy stretching guidelines.

- **Reach as far as you can.** Don't feel you have to touch your toes or bend over backward. For any stretch, reach as far as you can until you feel a slight tension in your muscle. If you feel pain or a burning sensation, on the other hand, you've gone too deep. Ease back until the pain goes away.

- **Hold it for at least 30 seconds.** Do each stretch for this long, and you'll only need to do it once. A whole minute may be in order if your muscle is really tight. Time yourself with a stopwatch at first to get the feel of how long this is. If you really enjoy stretching and feel you need it, repeat each stretch as many as three to five times.

- **Feel at ease and breathe.** This session is not a workout for your lungs, so breathe as you normally would. You're not supposed to clench your muscles, either. Relax every muscle except the ones you're stretching at the moment.

■ **Do not bounce.** No matter what your gym teacher taught you in high school, do not bounce when you stretch. You risk injury by doing it, and it may even make you less flexible.

Stretching's most dangerous list

The President's Council on Physical Fitness and Sports had your health in mind when it included these exercises in its list of most dangerous stretches.

■ **Yoga plow.** This stretch involves lying on your back and kicking your legs over the top of your head to the floor. It could cause serious neck damage if you have arthritis or osteoporosis.

■ **Neck circles.** Whipping your neck around quickly can hurt your neck and even your backbone. Do slow head tilts instead. (See page 142.)

■ **Toe touches.** Whether standing or sitting, these are never a good idea when done quickly. Focus on doing a slow, gradual stretch, and don't worry about reaching your toes.

■ **Hurdler stretch.** Sit with one leg straight out and the other bent behind you? Talk about dangerous for your knees! It's better to keep your bent leg in front of you. (See hamstring stretch on the next page.)

Limber up with safe stretches

Here are more than 10 stretching routines that will take 10 minutes a day or less. They will show you that getting fit is easier than you think. Some of these stretches may get rid of a swayback or potbelly. Others are easy and helpful ways to alleviate neck and back pain. By stretching regularly, your body will feel more relaxed and ready to take on everyday tasks.

LEGS **Hamstring stretch**

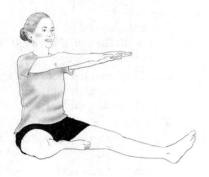

1. Sit up on the floor or in your bed.
2. Extend your left leg. Fold in your right leg so its foot points toward your right knee.
3. Lean forward, reaching your arms above your legs and leaving your back straight. Don't over-reach to touch your toes. Hold for 15 to 20 seconds.
4. Extend your right leg, fold your left, and repeat.

LEGS **Butterfly stretch**

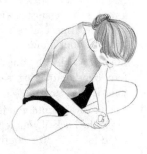

1. Sit with your feet touch-ing in front of you.
2. Hold your feet, leaning your elbows into the inside of your knees.
3. Push down gently on your knees until you feel a stretch in your groin. Hold for 5 seconds.

LEGS Thigh stretch

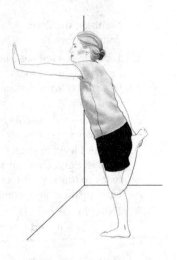

1. Stand facing a wall at arm's length. Place your left hand on it for support.
2. Lift up your left foot behind you, and grab it with your right hand.
3. Pull your left foot toward your buttocks, and hold for 30 seconds.
4. Let go of your left foot, switch hands and feet, and repeat with your right leg.

LEGS Calf stretch

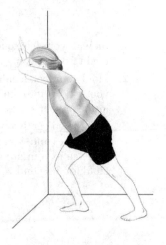

1. Stand about a foot away from a wall. Lean against it with your forearms, and rest your head on your hands.
2. Step forward with your right foot, bending that leg. Keep your left leg straight.
3. Lean forward until you feel a tug in the back of your left leg. Hold for 15 to 30 seconds.
4. Switch legs and repeat.

BACK Knee-to-chest stretch

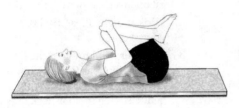

1. Lie on your back on the floor or in your bed.
2. Fold your legs on top of you so your knees touch your chest.
3. Grab your knees, and pull them down until you feel a stretch in your lower back. Hold for 30 seconds.

BACK Pelvic tilt

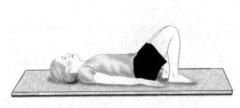

1. Lie on your back on the floor or in your bed.
2. Bend your knees, and plant your feet about one foot away from your buttocks.
3. Press the small of your back toward the floor, and tighten your abdominal muscles. Use your hips, not your legs. Hold for 5 seconds, then relax.

NECK **Head tilt**

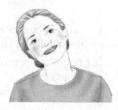

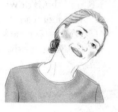

1. Sit up in a chair or in your bed.
2. Look straight ahead. Relax your shoulders.
3. Tilt your head to the right, leaning your ear toward your shoulder. When you feel a gentle stretch in your neck, hold for 10 seconds.
4. Straighten your head, then repeat to the left side.

NECK **Shoulder roll**

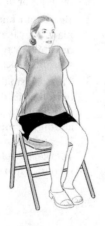

1. Sit in a chair or your bed with your arms at your sides.
2. Shrug your shoulders upward without bending your elbows.
3. Rotate your shoulders forward in a circle. Then rotate them backward.
4. Repeat each direction at least five times, making each circle bigger than the last.

UPPER BODY **Over-the-head shoulder stretch**

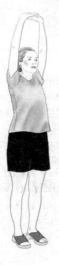

1. Stand up, or sit up in a chair or in bed.
2. Reach your arms over your head as far as they can go, and interlace your fingers.
3. Turn your palms upward. Gently push your arms back and up. Hold for 15 seconds.

UPPER BODY **Upper body twist**

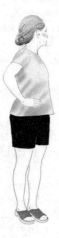

1. Stand up and place your hands on your hips.
2. Twist your upper body to the left as far as it can go, leaving your legs facing forward. Hold for 5 seconds.
3. Repeat to the right.

UPPER BODY Arm twist

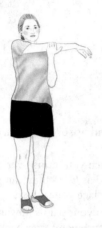

1. Sit or stand up.
2. Reach your right arm across your chest in front of your left shoulder.
3. Place your left hand on your right elbow and gently push. You'll feel a stretch in the back of your shoulder. Hold.
4. Switch arms and repeat.

UPPER BODY Shoulder rotation

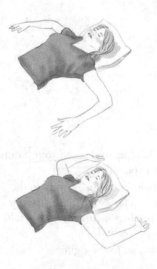

1. Lie on the floor or in your bed with a pillow beneath your head. If you have back problems, put a rolled towel underneath your knees.
2. Lay your arms out perpendicular to your body, and bend them up at the elbows so they look like goalposts.
3. Rotate your arms forward, moving your hands to the floor near your waist. Hold for 20 to 30 seconds.
4. Rotate your forearms up and then backward, moving your hands toward the floor near your head. Hold.

Walking: step out and shape up

8

Enjoy the slow, sure way to fitness

Walking doesn't require any special talent or training – you just do it without thinking. Yet if you put a little extra time and effort into it each day, just look at the results. You lose weight, have more energy, lower your blood pressure and cholesterol, think more clearly, have less anxiety, and sleep a whole lot better. And that's just the beginning.

Benefits like these have turned walking into one of the most popular fitness activities ever. People tend to give up on most exercise programs after the first big push, but walkers are more like the Energizer Bunny – they just keep on going. That's because they discover it is a steady, sure way to health and fitness. They don't stop when they get older, either. More men over 65 are regular walkers than in any other age group. For many people, a daily walk has become their ticket to a longer, healthier, more enjoyable life.

> **Famous walkers throughout history include Harry Truman, noted for his morning presidential walks, and writers Emerson and Thoreau, who walked for inspiration.**

Want more reasons to walk? Try these five and see if they don't persuade you to put on your walking shoes right now.

- You can walk just about any time you're in the mood. You don't have to make a reservation, change clothes, or wait for others to join you.

- You're less likely to get hurt than with other activities. Walking is low impact, so you don't have the stress on your joints that leads to blown-out knees, sprained ankles, and bad backs. Other health risks are almost zero because it's less strenuous than most activities.

- You can afford it – there are no clubs to join or expensive equipment to buy. All you really need is a pair of sturdy shoes.

- You can adjust your walking schedule around your other activities. If you need a break or have a few spare minutes, take a walk.

- You can do it anywhere – in your own neighborhood or local park, while you're shopping, even when you're out-of-town. If the weather is bad and you don't want to dress for it, walk indoors.

You may be one of the millions of couch potatoes who think they should get more exercise but aren't doing anything about it. Maybe you just want to feel better. Either way, take a few steps in the right direction, and start walking your way to fitness. What could be easier?

Just dust off your old sneakers – or better yet invest in a new pair (see buying advice later in this chapter) – and get up and go. Take your spouse or a friend for some quality time of fun and fitness. Before long, you'll be keeping up with the best of them and reaping the benefits of the walking fitness phenomenon.

Easy ways to get motivated

Before you start, get an OK from your doctor if you're at risk for heart disease, diabetes, or other serious health problems. It's not a bad idea to check anyway, especially if you're a man over age 40 or a woman over 50 and plan to make a big jump in the amount of your activity.

Next, make a commitment. Walking won't help much if you don't do it regularly, so find the motivation to stick with it. Come up with reasons why exercising is important to you. Reasons like:

- You'll be able to walk up the stairs without huffing and puffing.

- Attractive clothes will look good on you.

- You'll sleep better and be more relaxed and energetic.

- It will give you the confident air that fit people have.

- It will help you avoid health problems like colon cancer, heart attacks, and diabetes.

Write down your own reasons, and put the list on the refrigerator to remind you why walking is important to you, because sticking to the program may be a struggle at first. To get through the first few weeks, tell your plans to family and friends. You'll be embarrassed if you don't follow through, and they can encourage you and praise your progress when you keep going.

If you think you may get bored, deal with it ahead of time. Try these ideas to make your walks more interesting:

- Have a destination such as a coffee shop, post office, or library.

- Go where you can enjoy window shopping while you walk.

- Use your time for planning your day or just relaxing and thinking.

- Take along your dog, someone else's dog, or a friend or family member for company.

- Choose alternate routes each day. Get adventurous and explore new neighborhoods.

Once you've decided why you're going to walk, decide when – every morning, every evening, every other afternoon – and write it down on your calendar. You may have to make some choices, like cutting out a half-hour of TV or getting up an hour earlier in the morning. But scheduling it in writing shows you're serious about fitting it into your daily life.

To walk or run?

Some people think walking is too easy to be decent exercise, but others believe you can have "gain without pain" and that running and jogging are too hard on your body.

"I gave up running as a primary exercise in my 30s when I saw what it did to the knees and backs of my friends," says 51-year-old Frank Garver.

The fact is, you burn just as many calories per mile walking as you do running. It just takes longer – 20 minutes to walk a mile versus eight or 10 minutes to jog it. And a Harvard study found that walking protects you from heart problems just as much as more vigorous and challenging exercise.

Since it's also true that walkers suffer fewer injuries, you may as well walk if you have the time. It's important, though, to walk briskly. You won't get much of either conditioning or weight loss unless you raise your heart rate.

It's best to do at least 30 minutes of exercise at a time, but if shorter walks fit your schedule better, fine. Sometimes people who take several short walks each day stay with it better than those who do one long one. You'll still get a lot of benefit from a number of short sessions.

Where should you walk? Anywhere your heart desires. That's the beauty of this type of exercise. Of course, you want to make sure it's a safe area, and pleasant surroundings wouldn't hurt, either.

If you prefer the outdoors, you can walk on streets and sidewalks, in parks, or on trails built especially for walking. If you want a smooth, level surface, look for a school with an athletic track. In cities like Reston, Va., and Peachtree City, Ga., golf carts are a way of life, and you can walk on miles and miles of cart paths. Some places also have bicycle trails you can use.

Pamper your feet with proper shoes

Almost any shoes will work for walking, but if you walk a lot, you may want to invest in a supportive walking shoe. Use these tips when shopping.

- Pick sturdy shoes that fit well and are comfortable. You should not need to break them in.

- Walking shoes should be lightweight, bend at the ball of your foot, and have ample room in the toe area. The heel should be at least a half-inch higher than the sole so you won't overstretch your Achilles tendon.

- You can walk in running shoes, which are generally lighter, heavier cushioned, and more expensive. Many low-priced shoes are just as good, though.

- Try on shoes late in the day when your feet are the largest. Take a pair of socks you wear for walking.

- If you walk a lot, your shoes may wear out in just less than a year. Sometimes you can extend their life with new insoles. Try rough-textured insoles — they make your foot more sensitive, which some think helps you adjust your balance and gait to avoid injury.

Just be careful when you're sharing space with vehicles. Remember, it's hard for cars to avoid people in the street, and it's hard to hear golf carts and bicycles coming up behind you.

To walk indoors, go to large stores, shopping malls, or use the treadmills at gyms and other athletic facilities. You can even go from room to room in your own home. In downtown Minneapolis and other cold-weather cities, you can walk in enclosed skyways built above the streets between buildings.

As long as you're walking, think about simple ways you can add steps to your daily routine. For example:

- Park farther away in parking lots.

- Walk while you're on the telephone and during TV commercials.

- Go inside instead of taking the drive-through.

- Take the stairs instead of the elevator.

Start slow to stay positive

Don't expect to go full speed when you first start walking. Depending on the shape you're in, you may only be able to walk five or 10 minutes at a time. Be patient, and don't get discouraged. As your conditioning improves, you'll be surprised how much more you can do. To gradually build up strength, walk at least three times a week – five or six is better.

Walking is a good workout for your heart, lungs, and legs, but it's not a complete exercise program, and your other muscles can get stiff and tight. It helps to do some slow stretches before you walk. Many experts recommend you walk slowly for a few minutes to warm up before you stretch. You're less likely to get injured that way. It's important to stretch after walking also to cut down on aches and soreness the next day.

Dress to stay dry and comfortable, and use layers you can take off as you warm up. Bright colors are more visible, and reflective material is a must if you walk at dusk or dawn.

Look in the *Superstar stretches* chapter for the following stretches focusing on your legs and back. You should include these in your warmup routine.

- The calf stretch, thigh stretch, and hamstring stretch for the muscles in your legs.

- The torso twist, knee-to-chest stretch, and pelvic tilt for your back.

Others to try:

- A variation on the knee-to-chest stretch called the knee pull. Lean your back against a wall and pull one knee at a time to your chest for 10 seconds. This helps both your back and your hamstrings.

- Side reaches to stretch your back and side muscles. With one hand on your hip, reach the other arm over your head and to the opposite side. Try not to lean forward. Then switch to the other side.

After stretching, try to walk for 15 or 20 minutes. Go slower the first and last five minutes to warm up and cool down. Don't be concerned about how far you go – the pace and time spent are what's important.

When you first start, your target heart rate should only be around 50 or 60 percent of maximum. If you're not in very good shape, it won't take much to get there. To find out your heart rate and your target heart rate, refer to the chapter *Exercise: the secret to staying young.*

If you walk a mile in 20 minutes, you're going 3 miles per hour (mph), which is a low-end moderate pace. Don't worry if you're only doing 2 or 2 1/2 mph, though. It's your exertion level that's important. Don't overdo it. As your stamina improves, you will naturally speed up just to maintain your heart rate.

Step up the pace to feel fabulous

You may feel good enough to start out with 20-minute sessions, but if not, that's all right. Just pick a starting point and keep going farther and faster until you get where you want to be. Stick to your starting pace for a week and then start walking a little longer.

Make a 20-minute walk your first goal. That's about how long it takes to start getting real endurance benefits from sustained exercise. A good rule of thumb is to step it up about 10 percent a week. The following chart shows a schedule to get from 15 minutes to 45 minutes in about three months. This program works best when you're walking about five days a week. If you're doing less than three days a week, you should increase your time more slowly.

Walking plan: 45 minutes in 12 weeks

	Warm Up	Brisk Walk	Cool Down	Total Time
WEEK 1	5 min	5 min	5 min	15 min
WEEK 2	5 min	7 min	5 min	17 min
WEEK 3	5 min	9 min	5 min	19 min
WEEK 4	5 min	11 min	5 min	21 min
WEEK 5	5 min	13 min	5 min	23 min
WEEK 6	5 min	15 min	5 min	25 min
WEEK 7	5 min	18 min	5 min	28 min
WEEK 8	5 min	21 min	5 min	31 min
WEEK 9	5 min	24 min	5 min	34 min
WEEK 10	5 min	27 min	5 min	37 min
WEEK 11	5 min	31 min	5 min	41 min
WEEK 12	5 min	35 min	5 min	45 min

So far, you've been working to build up your walking time, but as you get into better shape, you can also raise your exertion level. Walk faster to boost your heartbeat a little more. Just don't increase both your speed and walking time during the same workout. Do one first and the other a day or two later. Make it your next goal to do three miles in 45 minutes – a 4-mph pace – and then keep going until you top out with a heart rate around 75 percent of maximum.

A brisk pace is important. If you're not sweating and breathing harder than normal, you're not getting a good workout. Don't stroll or saunter, but don't go too fast either, or you'll wear out too soon. Use the "talk test" to find the right pace – slow down if you can't carry on a conversation while you walk.

How long and how hard you walk is much more meaningful than how far you walk. At the top of the list, though, is how often you walk. If you don't walk regularly, you won't see steady improvement, and you can even lose ground. Walk at least three times a week to maintain a general level of fitness. Walk more often if you want to lose weight or raise your endurance level. But always schedule at least one day of rest per week. Your body needs some "down time" to recover.

Good technique is also important. When you walk:

- Keep your chin up, your shoulders back, and your belly flat.

- Take long, easy strides and land on your heel, rolling forward to the ball of your foot and pushing off from the toe.

- Breathe deeply and let your arms swing naturally.

- Lean forward a little when going fast or up and down hills.

Variety: the key to banishing boredom

Once you reach a fitness level you're happy with, you have a choice – continue at your current pace or take on a bigger challenge. If boredom is a problem, you need to shake up your routine a little. Try walking at different paces – some fast, some slow – during your workout. Add some hills to your route. You'll work harder going up and get a little relief going down. Stay indoors one day and go outdoors the next. Or try different types of walking like the ones below.

Power up your heart and lungs

Once your workout becomes second nature, you may want to raise the challenge with power walking. It's not as intense as racewalking, where you compete to see who walks fastest, but it's a good way to challenge your body to do even more than it's used to. Power walking won't help you lose any more weight per mile, but it will do wonders for your heart and lungs.

The first thing to keep in mind is that you walk much faster. You need to take shorter steps and keep a smooth stride. Next, you add more ambitious arm movements. As you walk faster, pump your arms higher – to chest or neck level. Working your arms is just as good as working your legs, so now you're doing double-duty.

Carrying additional weight will boost your calorie burn. You can supplement your own weight in the following ways if you're not prone to back or joint injuries.

- **Hand weights.** Carrying small dumbbells while you work your arms is like doing curls – one repetition per stride. Don't use weights heavier than 2 pounds, though – you could strain your shoulders.

- **Weighted gloves.** You don't have to grip these weights, which means more relaxed arms and shoulders. Plus you can't drop them.

- **Weight vest.** This is more expensive, but you can carry more weight and distribute the load to both your upper- and lower-body muscles.

Another way to supplement your power walking is to use poles or walking sticks. Moving the poles along with your feet makes your arms work more and gives your heart a better workout. Since they help support you, you don't feel like you're working any harder. Be sure to use them, though – it doesn't do much good to just carry them.

You can also change the surface you walk on. Walking through grass or soft dirt is tougher than cruising along on the pavement. Combine great exercise with a great vacation by going to California or Cancun or somewhere else with beautiful beaches. Walking in the sand will burn a lot more calories.

Rev up your motor with a treadmill

If you have trouble getting out the door, a treadmill may be just what you need. When you own a treadmill, it's right there reminding you of that appointment with yourself, and it's harder to come up with excuses to avoid your workout. It may be just the ticket if you or your doctor believes you need to exercise, and you don't quite have the enthusiasm to stay with it.

That's how it worked with Bill Morris, 61, whose doctor told him to get more serious about exercising after his blood pressure shot up to 186/92. Bill put himself on a regular treadmill schedule, lost 20 pounds, and dropped his blood pressure to 110/58.

"My doctor said the reduced blood pressure was probably due as much to weight loss as it was to exercise," he says. "But then, I wouldn't have lost the weight without walking on the treadmill. You've got to find a way to make walking a regular, rarely missed appointment with yourself. If I put it off, something always gets in the way."

Like Bill, many people prefer the controlled environment of walking indoors. You're out of the weather and can read, watch TV, or listen to music while you walk. That, in itself, makes your workout more interesting. You can also manage how hard you work by adjusting the speed and incline of your treadmill. Most are programmed to show time, distance, and calories, too, which helps you keep track of your progress. Seeing how many calories you've burned is a great incentive to keep moving! Higher-priced machines have heart-rate monitors and other sophisticated attachments that fine-tune your workout even more.

Because it's so easy to operate, you're more likely to stick with a treadmill than with other kinds of machines. It's no wonder it's the most popular exercise machine. It's also the best for getting the most exercise, according to a laboratory study at the Medical College of Wisconsin. Researchers there compared six kinds of exercise machines. The treadmill gave more benefit for the effort than stair steppers and cross-country skiing machines. Rowing machines and two kinds of indoor cycles gave the least.

Top-notch treadmill-buying tips

You can spend from $300 to more than $3,000 on a treadmill, so choose carefully. If you're only using it for walking, a less durable — and less expensive— one will probably do just fine.

Wear your walking shoes so you can try it out at the store. Is the belt long and wide enough for your stride? Are the handrails in the right position to grip and keep your balance? Does it feel solid and sturdy? Are the monitors and controls easy to reach and read?

The motor should be rated at least two horsepower continuous — not peak — duty for longevity. It should have at least a two-ply belt and a sturdy deck. Make sure it's not too noisy.

Take a tape measure and see if it will fit in the space you have for it. Will it fold up for storage? If so, try it in the store to see if you can manage it. And don't forget to ask about warranty and service.

Find fun and fitness on the trail

To get more out of your outdoor walks, try taking a hike. Get into the woods or out in the country, and walk the trails instead of the sidewalks. The more rugged terrain requires more exertion, and you'll probably discover muscles you never knew you had.

Lots of parks and preserves feature hiking trails that range from easy walks to expert climbs. Check out the closest national, state, county, or even city park. Wherever you go, the beauty and peacefulness of nature will be an added bonus to the exercise you get.

Some tips for new hikers:

- Plan to go about half the distance you usually walk. Rough ground, abrupt inclines, and obstacles like trees and rocks will give you a more challenging workout than you're used to.

- At first, just go down a trail a certain distance and then turn around and come back. That way, you'll have a better idea where you are and how long you've been gone. Later on you can graduate to circle routes that bring you back to the starting point.

- Pay extra attention to your shoes when hiking. It's easy to get blisters and chaffing on uneven surfaces with shoes that don't fit well. You can probably use your regular walking shoes, but make sure they have good ankle support. Consider hiking boots if you will be out more than two or three hours.

- For longer hikes, you'll want to take maps, water bottles, food, and various equipment with you. Carry them in a fanny pack or a small day pack – the extra weight will add to your exercise.

- Take along a walking stick for better balance and support on the trail.

The ultimate "walk in the park" is overnight backpacking – carrying food, tents, and sleeping bags. The added weight and longer time spent hiking means more exercise. It also requires better conditioning before you start, but you can do it if you gradually work yourself into shape.

The payoff is the exhilaration that comes from demanding exercise and the satisfaction of getting somewhere you thought you couldn't go. So, for a simple, easy exercise program, start walking. And, whether it takes you to the sidewalks, the gym, or the woods, you'll feel better and have a good time getting there. Happy trails!

The "Quick" way to better health

Lorette Quick is 77 years old and a familiar sight in Senoia, Ga., even though she's lost more than 100 pounds. You'll see her walking three times a day – from her house on the edge of town to the other side of town and back – for a daily total of about 10 miles.

She started walking seven years ago after the death of her husband.

"My husband was real sick and I didn't get out of the house for a long time," Lorette says. "He had 17 kinds of medicine and needed taking care of. I just couldn't leave. When he died, I weighed 260 pounds and I felt real bad. I had to do something."

So, a little like Forrest Gump, Lorette started walking. After a year or so, she only weighed 145 pounds and had a much brighter outlook on life. Now, she feels better and has none of the ailments people her age usually have.

She makes her first trip every morning right after breakfast. She goes again at lunchtime and once more in the evening. She stops and visits with people along the way and sometimes makes a side trip through the cemetery to tend her husband's grave.

"The scales got down to 145 and stayed there," she testifies. "I eat whatever I like, and my cholesterol and everything else is normal. I get a checkup every six months, and my doctor says there's nothing wrong with me."

Lorette mows her own yard – it's about half an acre so she uses a riding mower – and does alterations and other sewing for people in town. Walking is her passion, though.

"When it's raining or something and I can't walk, I feel bad, can't sleep at night," she says. "Even when it does rain, I try to find time to walk in between the showers."

12 ways to walk your way to perfect health

Walking is an easy, satisfying way to exercise that you can do any place at any time. Follow these suggestions to make walking a permanent part of your healthy lifestyle.

- Walk alone, for meditation and to clear your mind.

- Go with a partner on a regular schedule.

- Walk during lunch hours or breaks at work.

- Take long sightseeing walks while on vacation.

- Go sightseeing in your own town.

- Go shopping downtown or at the mall.

- Visit a park.

- Explore hiking trails.

- Take advantage of golf cart paths or bicycle trails.

- Walk on a treadmill at home or the gym.

- Walk your dog, or push a baby carriage.

- Walk instead of driving anywhere within half a mile.

Aerobics: a body-boosting workout

Improve your fitness 3 ways

The beauty of regular, low-impact aerobic exercise is that you can reap big rewards with relatively little time and effort – especially if you've been a couch potato. All forms of this type of exercise concentrate on fitness and endurance more than strength. And if you stick to low-impact, activities without a lot of jarring and strain on your joints, there's less wear and tear on your body.

By definition, aerobic exercise uses the oxygen you breathe to produce energy and allow you to work out for a long period of time. Some aerobic activities are jogging, dancing, bicycling, skating, swimming, and even shoveling and mowing.

Walking, of course, is the quickest and easiest way to start an aerobic program, but if you're looking for greater variety or a bigger challenge, there are plenty of other aerobic exercises you can do – and have fun at the same time. Some – like bicycling yourself into shape for a road race – involve pushing yourself harder and farther. Some – like water and step aerobics – might mean enrolling in a class. But all aerobic activities, if done regularly, will improve your overall fitness.

Strengthen your heart and lungs

An aerobic exercise raises your heart rate and keeps it up – at around 60 to 85 percent of your heart rate maximum. This increases the amount of oxygen your body delivers to your muscles. The more oxygen they have, the longer they can work without fatiguing. Therefore, aerobic exercise strengthens your heart and increases your lungs' ability to gather oxygen, making the whole system more efficient.

Good aerobic activity is continuous, repetitive, and usually rhythmic. It works large muscles at a pace that uses oxygen about as fast as you take it in. When this happens, you give your muscles a constant bath of fresh oxygen while your heart and lungs get a good workout. As they become stronger, you are able to exercise longer and harder with less effort. The result: you gain endurance and muscle tone.

Burn away fat calories

Aerobic exercise is great for weight loss, too. It speeds up your metabolism, which stimulates the fat-burning process. Your metabolism continues at a faster pace even after you've stopped exercising, so the better you condition your aerobic system, the more fat you use up.

What is anaerobic exercise?

Imagine the opposite of aerobic exercise, and you've got anaerobic exercise. It refers to a short burst of vigorous activity – like sprinting, jumping, or lifting weights.

This type of exercise is so demanding, it pushes your heart rate above 85 percent of the maximum level. When this happens, your muscles need more energy than your oxygen supply creates through burning fat. So, your body begins to burn stored carbohydrates and protein calories.

That's why anaerobic activities may be helpful for building muscle mass but they won't help you lose weight.

Other anaerobic activities include baseball, tennis, and washing windows.

That's why Jo Bauer, 57, started participating in a water aerobics program several years ago. "My cholesterol was getting high and I wanted to lose weight," she explains. "In the last eight years, I've lost almost 40 pounds."

Jo takes two water aerobics classes a week, does land aerobics, some weight training, and walks every morning.

She likes water aerobics because you encounter resistance in every direction. "It's not like lifting a weight and then putting it back down," she says. "There are more muscles involved."

Her advice is to find a place to exercise that's convenient and then make it a part of your regular routine.

Check up before you work out

You want to exercise wisely and safely. So plan a visit to your doctor before you start any type of activity if you:

■ have heart disease risk factors such as age, heredity, smoking, diabetes, inactivity, etc.

■ have ever been told you have a heart condition.

■ have high blood pressure or high cholesterol, or are taking medication for either.

■ ever experience chest pains, irregular heartbeats, or dizziness.

■ suffer from bone or joint problems, or some other chronic health problem.

Even if you're perfectly healthy, you should also check with the doctor if you're a man over 40 or a woman over 50 and plan to begin exercising more vigorously than usual.

Lower the pressure

When your heart and lungs are in condition, not only will you feel better, but you're more likely to avoid heart problems, high blood pressure, obesity, depression, diabetes, and a host of other life-shortening ills.

And don't worry about exercise aggravating your high blood pressure. A Princeton University report recommends aerobic exercise for both prevention and treatment of high blood pressure.

A blood pressure reading of 120/80 used to be cause for celebration. But the National Heart, Lung, and Blood Institute (NHLBI) now says if your systolic pressure (the top number) is between 120 and 139 and your diastolic pressure (the bottom number) is between 80 and 89, you are considered "pre-hypertensive."

This means you are at risk for developing full-blown hypertension, or high blood pressure. According to experts at the NHLBI, lifestyle changes – like exercise and weight loss – are the best ways to treat this new risk category. Residents of a Maryland retirement community, all in their 80s, proved this true recently.

Regular, moderate exercise that improves your heart and lung fitness is best for lowering blood pressure. Start slow, and gradually increase the effort and time spent on your workout.

For six months, they walked on treadmills or rode exercise bikes for 30 minutes, two or three times a week. By exercising safely under their doctor's supervision, all increased their ability to use oxygen while exercising – a measurement of physical fitness. And they lowered their blood pressure.

Here are some fun-to-do low-impact aerobic ideas that will have you fit in no time.

Step up to a healthier body

Back in 1870, the lighthouse keeper for the Cape Hatteras Light Station in North Carolina may have invented step aerobics. At that time, the lighthouse contained 18 oil-burning lamps that had to be lit every night and turned off every morning. Climbing the 268 cast-iron steps twice a day was certainly excellent aerobic exercise.

In fact, step training classes and videos have been a popular form of aerobic exercise only since the late 1980s, but the principle of lifting your own body weight to improve cardiovascular fitness is not new. When you ran up and down the bleachers in junior high gym class, you were performing a time-honored conditioning drill.

You also know that climbing the staircase in your home – like going to the top of the Hatteras Light Station (it still doesn't have an elevator, by the way) – takes extra energy. As a matter of fact, the simplest way to get started on step aerobics is to go up and down your stairs at home.

Another way is to use the bottom stair as a platform. Just step up onto it and back down. You could also buy a stair-climber exercise machine.

If you want something a little more structured, try a step aerobics class or buy a video to use at home. You'll learn how to properly step onto and off of a low bench or platform. A class leader or instructor demonstrates the movements to music and keeps the routine going.

Step aerobics is an ideal workout because you get the cardiovascular benefits of running but the lower joint-stress of walking. It uses the large muscles in your legs and is rhythmic and repetitive – all essentials of aerobic exercise. There's also an element of strength training involved. By raising and lowering the weight of your body, you're building muscles, too.

Once you get your footwork down, you can boost the intensity of your workout by adding arm movements. Just don't work your arms above shoulder level for any length of time since this can hurt your shoulders. Rather, change frequently from low- to mid- to high-range movements.

Most experts do not recommend you use hand weights while you are step training. You're more likely to damage your joints and they don't add much benefit.

Low and slow is best for beginners

Be careful about the intensity of your step aerobic workout, especially when you are just starting out. People who have been at it a while often enjoy the challenge of fancy steps, fast music, and tall benches. If you try to keep up with them in the beginning, you can become discouraged and give up altogether. You may even hurt yourself if the workout is too extreme.

In fact, when you're doing step aerobics, faster is not necessarily better. Experts say music with about 122 beats per minute keeps you within your target training zone. Going faster not only compromises your control and safety but can easily turn your workout into more stressful high-impact, anaerobic exercise.

Be careful of power moves — those that involve hopping, jumping, and lunging. While they make you work harder, they are also higher impact and increase the stress on your joints and your risk of injury.

Tips for successful stepping

■ Start out with a bench that's only about four inches high – when you haven't been exercising regularly, it doesn't take much to elevate your heart rate. As you get better with your footwork and conditioning, raise the step to boost your workout.

■ When you do graduate to a taller bench, don't ever choose one that makes you step so high you have to bend your knees more than 90 degrees. With your foot resting on the platform, your hip should still be higher than your knee. And if you have knee problems, consult your doctor before doing any step training.

■ Use good posture – head and chest up, abdominal muscles lightly contracted, and buttocks tucked under your hips.

■ Watch the platform when stepping up to make sure you get your entire foot on it. Letting your heel hang over the edge invites Achilles tendon problems.

■ Step softly and quietly to avoid stress on your ankles and knees.

■ Stay close to the platform when stepping down and let your heel touch the floor to help absorb the impact.

■ The leg that begins the step pattern is called the leading leg and it receives the most stress. For that reason, don't lead with the same leg for more than one minute.

■ You can change the intensity of your workout by moving faster or stepping higher. However, if you're in a class with faster music, keep the platform low. If the music is slow, raise the platform. Don't increase both at the same time.

Water exercise works wonders

The water is a terrific place for fitness. Its buoyancy reduces the stress on your weight-bearing joints by as much as 90 percent – cutting down on muscle soreness and injury. Yet water provides the resistance needed to develop a strong heart and lungs. This combination can certainly make you feel better physically, but it gives you a mental boost, too.

"There is a freedom that cannot be gotten any other way," explains Dr. Bill Best, retired swimming coach and professor of physical education and health at Berea College in Kentucky. "It's the closest thing we have to weightlessness. In fact, this is how the astronauts trained."

Splash away stiffness with water aerobics

Water aerobics is probably the ultimate low-impact exercise. It's sometimes the only way for certain people to exercise – pregnant women, the elderly or overweight, people with arthritis, or those recovering from surgery or injury. But anyone can benefit.

"Water aerobics is not a strength conditioning type of exercise," says Cajen Rhodes, program director for a city Parks and Recreation pool. "It works on range of motion and on cardiovascular. It allows people to do things that they might not be able to do on land."

"A lot of people think it's land aerobics in the water," he says, "but it's not. You're a lot lighter in the water, so you can do full motion – a full range of pull-ups and things like that. In land aerobics, you're working under your own body weight. In water, you're working against the water's resistance. They use different types of movements, requiring different types of exercises. If you simply do land aerobics under the water it can definitely be counterproductive."

Rhodes also says water exercise is good for general aches and pains. "As you get older, your muscles get tighter, your legs and back get stiffer. The exercise helps keep you loose, keep you limber. It helps people – especially older people – in their day-to-day activities."

The best way to take advantage of water aerobics, even if you have your own pool, is to enroll in a class. You can find them through local recreation departments, the YMCA or YWCA, or fitness clubs and gyms. Many country club, neighborhood, and subdivision pools also offer classes.

"In a class, you're under the direct supervision of a qualified instructor who can give you the exercises you need to know," says Rhodes. "They serve as motivators who can get you on the right track and get you the best results."

General water aerobics classes spend about 10 minutes stretching and then do routines with dumbbells, belts, and ankle straps that serve as both flotation and resistance devices. They also walk and run in the water and do exercises while suspended in the water.

Rhodes' pool has special classes just for those with arthritis. "We keep the water warmer, which tends to be more therapeutic to our classes. It loosens up their muscles and ligaments and they're able to stretch easier," he says, "They spend the majority of their time just stretching – in different positions and doing different types of movements under the water. After they've been in the water for a while, they always feel better."

Water exercise eases arthritis pain

Dolores Regan has always exercised regularly, but because of back surgery and arthritis, she switched about five years ago from floor exercises and yoga to water aerobics. Now, at 72, she goes to a class three times a week and walks on her off days.

"Walking is a different type of thing," Dolores says, "because you're not using your arms. We do water exercises with our arms, hands, neck, legs, and feet. The walking is good, but I get more with the water exercises."

Dolores experiences a lot of pain and numbness in her arms and hands. "We do stretching and toning – very slowly," she explains. "And we use weights and bands and we do wall exercises in the water. I find when I do these things, my arms don't hurt as badly." She also says the exercise prevents stiffness.

Dolores credits her long-term activity with keeping her healthy. "When I had my back done, the therapist said he believed all the exercising I did prior to the operation helped me recuperate a lot quicker and better," she says. "I was supposed to go into rehab for three weeks, but they sent me straight home."

Dive into aerobic fitness

If you want a more solitary water exercise and don't need the structure of a class, just go swimming.

"Any type of swimming is great exercise," says Rhodes. "When you're swimming laps, you're working pretty much every muscle in your body – cardiovascular and everything else."

"You can get a very good aerobic workout swimming," agrees Best. He has these tips for getting the most out of a swimming workout.

■ "Start with some good instruction," he says. "Learn some of the modern techniques, develop some passable strokes, and then you can swim at your own speed and eventually get faster and faster."

■ "Master to some degree the breaststroke, the backstroke, the crawl stroke and – if you're strong enough – the butterfly," he continues. "I know people in their 50s and early 60s that can still do the butterfly."

■ "Learn sculling movements. Sculling is a figure eight movement with the hands that is used extensively to stay afloat in synchronized swimming and aquatic art. It can be very rigorous."

But what if you haven't been in the water for a while and are hesitant to dive back in? Best, who taught all levels and ages of swimmers for 45 years, believes that learning how to float and then developing swimming strokes will build your confidence. "I still think it's better," he says, "to learn the strokes and overcome that fear of the water than go into the deep end with a flotation device on. It makes you more dependent on the flotation device." Don't worry if you flounder around some when you first start swimming. This actually gives you a good aerobic workout, too.

"Speed will come at whatever level you want and feel you can do," he explains. But if you're not interested in becoming a speed swimmer, be content with simply using the water as resistance. This will still get your heart and lungs pumping.

If you're already a pretty good swimmer and want to maintain or even boost your skills and fitness level, look into United States Masters Swimming (USMS). This national organization provides organized workouts, clinics, and competitions for adult swimmers. Local USMS committees arrange for their members to swim at local pools and often have full-time or volunteer coaches who help with individual workouts.

USMS programs vary from non-competitive to triathlete training. Find out how to join and other particulars by visiting its Web site at <www.usms.org>.

Tips for swimming success

Whether you decide to take an aerobics class or just swim for fitness, you'll want the right equipment, facility, and instruction.

- Purchase a swimming suit that fits well and doesn't inhibit your movements. It should be a comfortable, sturdy style.

- For swimming, a pair of goggles helps keep water and chemicals out of your eyes and improves your underwater vision.

- A swimming cap will protect your hair from sun and chemicals and keep it out of your eyes.

- Equipment like weights, kickboards, paddles, and flotation aids should be furnished as part of your class. After you learn to use them, you may decide you want your own.

- When choosing a place to swim, look around the facility to see if it is clean and well maintained. Is the water in the pool clear and sparkling? Does a city or county health inspector regularly check the chemical balance of the water? Is the staff friendly, helpful, and knowledgeable?

- Talk to the instructor before you sign up for a class, and explain what you're trying to accomplish with your exercise program. Ask if they can recommend a specific class to help you reach your objectives.

- If you are just beginning to swim, look for a good teacher, not a coach. "Not all swimming coaches are good teachers," cautions Best. "The characteristics that make them good coaches sometimes make them poor teachers. Teaching and training are quite different."

Bicycling: fun for life

In 1973, John Karras and Don Kaul, both writers for *The Des Moines Register*, decided to ride bicycles from one end of Iowa to the other – producing columns and articles for the newspaper along the way. They invited their readers to join them, and between 100 and 500 riders cycled in and out of the six-day ride.

The event was so successful that it turned into RAGBRAI – the Register's Annual Great Bicycle Ride Across Iowa – and now must limit the number of weeklong riders to 8,500. It has also inspired more than 40 similar rides around the country. Karras rode in 28 events and wrote stories about the trip and the towns they went through, traveling 450 to 500 miles, fighting hills, heat, humidity, and headwinds.

"I bought my first 10-speed bicycle in 1967 at age 37, and it changed my life," Karras recalls. "I had ridden some as a child and a lot the summers of my college years – all on an old one-speed, fat-tired bike. The 10-speed was a revelation. I thought I'd never have to pedal again."

"I talked my best friend into buying one and in a few years we had become touring cyclists, discovering that Iowa is incredibly beautiful from the seat of a bicycle. The more we rode the fitter we became. Neither of us had been athletes as young men," he says, "but the bikes changed all that."

Now 73 and retired in Colorado, Karras is no longer an official part of RAGBRAI, but he and his wife, Ann, still bike, hike, and ski.

"How fit am I?" Karras asks. "Compared to the general population of my age, very. Compared to the seniors in Summit County, maybe average or a little below. We live above 9,000 feet, which makes just about everything a little more difficult. Last year, for the first time since we moved here, we approached our old levels of fitness – we managed to ride about 1,500 miles."

Karras' story demonstrates the appeal bicycling has for many people – it's one of America's most popular activities and one of the best aerobic exercises. But you don't have to ride 4,000 miles a year – as Karras and his wife used to do – to get fun and fitness from your two-wheeler.

When you can't or don't want to cycle outdoors, try an exercise bike either at home or the gym. Enroll in a spinning class if you want a high-energy workout.

Simply pedal around your neighborhood, get your heart pumping a little faster for 20 or 30 minutes, and enjoy the local sights you never see from a car window.

If you are lucky, you can take a trail ride through nearby parks. Why not ride your bike to work, particularly if you live where traffic and parking are frustrating. If biking becomes a passion, consider a newer bike – they now come with up to 30 speeds – and venture into the country for day trips.

However you ride, you are steadily and continuously working your large lower-body muscles. This prompts your heart and lungs to carry more oxygen, increasing your overall fitness.

Ride a bike that's right for you

The first step in any cycling program is to find a bike. You could spend more than $1,000 for one, but it's smarter to start low and upgrade as you learn more about bikes and how you want to ride.

If you have one, dig out your old one-speed, fat-tired bike – or borrow one. Take a few rides to get the feel of it before you get serious about purchasing a new one. There are a lot of choices out there.

- **Road bikes.** Made for racing and riding on hard pavement, these bikes feature lightweight materials, skinny tires, and turned-down handlebars that allow the bent-over, aerodynamic posture of professional racers. It's the best kind of bike if you're going a long way, but watch out for the fancier racing bikes. They sacrifice durability and shock absorption for ultra-lightweight – and expensive – materials.

- **Mountain bikes.** These bikes – with their knobby tires and heavier frames – are made for rough terrain. They have flat handlebars so you sit upright, and lower gear ratios which make them slower but easier to pedal, especially going uphill.

- **Hybrid bikes.** Built for hard surfaces, hybrids are a cross between mountain bikes and road bikes. They have narrow, treaded tires and higher gears than mountain bikes. They include comfort bikes, which are heavy and have soft seats; and fitness bikes, which are fast and light. You don't have to bend over to ride either one.

- **Cruisers.** These look like the old Schwinns of the 1940s and 50s with large tires and comfortable seats. Most are one speed, but some may have as many as seven speeds. As the name implies, they're great for just cruising the neighborhood.

You can buy used bicycles through the want ads; or at garage sales, police auctions, and bike shops that take trade-ins. Look for a new bike at mass merchandise or large sporting goods stores and at bicycle specialty shops.

Whatever you buy, it's money well-spent to have your bike checked over and tuned-up by a qualified bike mechanic. The advantage of specialty shops is that they usually have mechanics on staff and often offer free tune-ups on bikes they sell.

Bike shops generally have more expensive but higher quality merchandise – meaning lighter, stronger materials, greater durability, and smoother-working moving parts. You'll also get advice on features you need and don't need, and help choosing the proper size bike, an important factor for enjoyable riding.

Gear up for safety and comfort

A helmet is the only additional piece of equipment you absolutely must have for bicycling. Regular clothing will do, as long as it allows freedom of movement and won't get tangled up in your bike chain. But don't be too embarrassed to get a pair of spandex biking shorts – most have built-in padding for your seat.

Other helpful equipment you should consider:

- Stiff-soled shoes work best for pedaling, and biking gloves help reduce vibration and protect your hands if you fall.

- A water bottle is vital if you ride for any length of time. One rule of thumb is to drink water every 15 minutes.

- Consider a mirror on your helmet if you're riding in traffic.

- Get a lock to secure your bike if you're going to leave it unattended.

- A basic repair kit that includes tire-patching material is handy. Or just take along a cell phone so you can call someone if you break down.

Before you start out, take a few minutes to familiarize yourself with your new bike – adjust the seat, test the brakes, and get the feel of the gear shifters. Begin with slow, comfortable rides of 15 to 30 minutes on flat ground. Progress to longer, faster rides and include hills as you get better and stronger.

"Starting bicycling is like starting any form of exercise," Karras says. "Ease into it. Otherwise it will be too painful to continue."

As you get into shape, you might decide you really like riding your bike and become a "touring cyclist" like Karras. As you discover how far you can go and how much you can see on your bike, you may even want to look into going on RAGBRAI or a similar event closer to home.

Pedal for fun and adventure

There are lots of cycling challenges you can take part in, including short or long treks organized by bike clubs and tour operators.

These range from Bike New York — a one-day, 42-mile ride through the five boroughs of New York City with 30,000 other cyclists — to the Big Ride Across America — a 48-day, 3,300-mile, cross-country expedition limited to 35 riders.

The National Bicycle Tour Directors Association's Web site at <www.nbtda.com> is a good place to explore the possibilities of these and other rides.

Grab a good time with more aerobic exercise

Walking, swimming, cycling, and stepping are some of the most common forms of aerobic exercise. But there are other ways you can have fun and get your fitness level up at the same time. Most require special settings and equipment, but all have an element of excitement.

If you like being around water, try rowing or canoeing – you can even take a fishing pole with you. If you live where there's snow, cross-country skiing and snowshoeing are better exercise than walking. If you don't have balance problems, ice-skating can be fun, too. Where there's no ice, try in-line skates.

Running, jogging, and jumping rope are higher impact ways to get your heart beating. Athletics like handball, racquetball, basketball, and soccer also provide good workouts. Be careful about playing too hard, though. Whenever your muscles need more oxygen than you're taking in, you've gone beyond aerobic conditioning into anaerobic exercise.

3 paths to better balance

10

Low-impact exercises are fun and healthy

Not everyone is made for high-level exercising. But you can become fit without bouncing around in a leotard, battering your joints. Forget all the huffing, puffing, lugging, lifting, and straining. Movement therapy is a gentle – yet effective – group of sports that include yoga, tai chi, and Pilates. Just don't be fooled by their mild manner. These activities can whip you into shape without breaking a sweat.

All three have ancient Eastern roots and are merely different interpretations of the same principle: keeping your body and mind in harmony naturally leads to better health.

It wasn't until recently that modern science confirmed the many physical benefits of yoga, tai chi, and Pilates. With them, you can improve your balance, flexibility, and strength – no matter what your age, weight, or fitness level.

No pain – but great gain

Yoga, tai chi, and Pilates are gentle enough for anyone to try. If you consider yourself in bad health or disabled in some way, you're a perfect candidate for these movement therapies. You can ease into the programs slowly and set your own pace. It's easy to stick with them and you'll see improvement quickly.

Here are just some of the benefits you will get from these soothing approaches to fitness.

■ When you were a child, tripping and falling meant just another minor scrape. But as you get older, taking a tumble can have serious and crippling effects. If your sense of balance is as bad as Humpty Dumpty's, these are the safest forms of exercise for you.

Just like the trick to growing tomatoes is to keep the main stalk strong, the trick to great balance is to keep your core muscles strong. The bands of muscle in your abdomen, lower back, and buttocks are the center of strength and control for the rest of your body.

All three examples of movement therapy are relatively stationary, but because they strengthen your core muscles, your balance will improve quickly – preventing falls – and you'll develop greater flexibility and strength. Soon you will be moving with confidence again.

■ Tai chi and yoga are especially recommended for people with arthritis. Gentle yoga can improve arthritis in your hands, for example, and tai chi's precise, flowing movements help keep your joints limber, relieve your pain, and keep you active.

■ The dance-like stretches, poses, and maneuvers within each of these movement therapies will gently strengthen and tone your body. Pilates is especially good as a strength-training workout.

■ Add yoga or Pilates to your exercise regimen if you need to improve your heart health.

■ In today's hectic world, it may be hard to squeeze an extra 30 minutes of exercise into your schedule – at least without feeling even more stress. The beautiful thing about movement therapy is that it combines stress relief with exercise, so you kill two birds with one stone.

All the activities – tai chi, yoga, and Pilates – are done slowly, with intense focus on proper breathing and posture. They all relax your body and calm your mind.

As you can see, you can boost your overall health with these joyful, health-giving movements.

Things to know before you give it a go

Just to be safe, make sure you take these precautions before starting any new exercise program.

■ Get your doctor's approval on your fitness plan, especially if you've badly injured your back, neck, knees, or shoulders in the past.

- The stretches, poses, and movements of these therapies should not hurt. If you feel pain, stop and check your technique before continuing.

- Pilates is the most intense of the three exercise forms. You may want to try one of the less strenuous programs first if you are out of shape.

- Be forewarned, you might get addicted to these calming sports.

Sidestep stiffness with yoga

You don't have to contort your body in order to benefit from yoga. Based on ancient health practices from India, yoga uses a series of gentle fixed poses and stretches to loosen your limbs and calm your mind. Today it's the darling of doctors searching for a way to keep the body and the mind fit into those golden years.

Yoga will change the way you think about aging. Because it increases your flexibility and aids breathing, you can practice it indefinitely. The famous Delaney sisters, Sadie and Bessie, were over 100 years old and still doing yoga six days a week before they died.

Enthusiasts agree that it is the perfect anti-stress exercise. No running, no sweating, no heavy weights. Yet, yoga is scientifically proven to relieve tension, reduce your cholesterol, and lower your blood pressure.

There are many different kinds of yoga. The most common is Hatha, which focuses on slow stretches, deep breathing, and meditation. Others include Bikram, which is often practiced within settings at temperatures over 80 degrees, and Ashtanga, a type requiring constant movement.

Get down to the basics

Here are some pointers to keep in mind before you begin yoga.

- You need very little gear for yoga – just comfortable, loose clothing and a mat to protect your back.

- Correct breathing technique is critical to a successful yoga workout. Follow the breathing instructions for each exercise exactly and always breathe through your nose.

- Start with some basic moves and concentrate on perfecting them before you move on to harder poses.

■ Never push a stretch to the point of pain. Never bounce or jerk.

■ Some of the more difficult poses could hurt your neck and back. Make sure you get proper instruction, and clear these exercises with your doctor first.

Here are a few poses to get you started.

YOGA Mountain pose

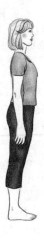

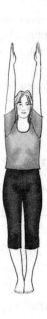

1. Stand tall, your feet together, your hands at your sides, and your weight evenly balanced.

2. Spread your toes apart and settle your feet firmly onto the floor.

3. Tuck you hips in, and puff your chest out just a bit.

4. Lengthen your neck by lifting the top of your head toward the ceiling.

5. Imagine a line running straight up through your body and out the top of your head.

6. Hold this pose for 5 to 10 slow, deep breaths.

7. Raise your arms over your head with your palms inward.

8. Breathe in deeply. Imagine the air coming up through your body, then going back down to your toes. Hold this pose for 5 to 10 breaths.

9. Lower your arms on an exhale and repeat 5 times.

YOGA Half warrior

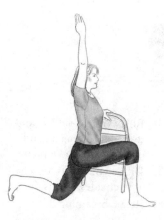

1. Place your right foot 3 to 4 feet in front of your body.

2. Drop your left knee gently to the floor so you are in a lunge position. Keep your right knee in line with your right ankle.

3. If you need to, hold on to a chair or table for balance, or place a blanket under your knee.

4. Keeping your back straight and your eyes forward, inhale and bring your arms straight up over your head. Place your palms together.

5. Hold for 4 or 5 deep breaths, then return to your starting position.

6. Repeat on the other side.

YOGA Easy cobra lift

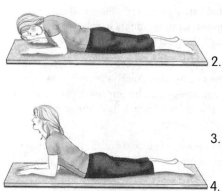

1. Lie down on your stomach. Place your elbows on the mat close to your body, and your palms flat on the mat near your head.

2. Without lifting your elbows off the floor, raise your chest up and out. Keep your hips and legs flat against the mat.

3. Don't tilt your head too far back. Look ahead and hold the pose for a few seconds.

4. Release, relax, and repeat twice more.

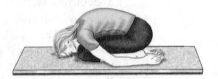

1. Assume a kneeling position with the tops of your feet against your mat.

2. Lower your buttocks down until they rest on your heels. If you have difficulty with this position, place a folded blanket between your calves and your buttocks.

3. Bend forward and drop your chest onto your thighs.

4. Relax your shoulders and rest your forehead gently on the mat or on a pillow.

5. Drape your arms loosely at your sides, palms up.

6. Relax, breathing deeply.

7. Hold for a minute or two.

8. Return very slowly to a sitting position.

Age gracefully with tai chi

Originally developed as a martial arts-style of self-defense, tai chi uses a series of postures and slow, continuous movements to relax and align your body. It has become through the years a form of exercise and personal development.

■ Tai chi is a fun and easy way to improve your balance by teaching you to be aware of your surroundings and by improving your muscle tone. Better balance means fewer falls. In fact, Tai chi can reduce your risk of falling by almost 50 percent.

■ Tai chi is one of the Chinese secrets of eternal youth. It relaxes your heart and your mind. Seniors who practiced it 30 minutes a day, four days a week for 12 weeks, reduced their blood pressure about as much as those in a more strenuous aerobic exercise program.

■ Don't give in to arthritis pain that makes motion painful. Tai chi is the alternative that can actually ease your pain. Dr. Paul Lam, a physician, a student of tai chi for over 30 years, and a world leader in the field of tai chi for health improvement, has developed a special program called Tai Chi for Arthritis. It's proven so helpful in easing pain and stiffness in arthritic joints, that it has been recognized by arthritis foundations around the world.

Tai chi is fun to do in a class, and easy enough to practice alone at home. It boosts your memory skills and relieves stress. If more vigorous forms of exercise are not for you, try this gentle "meditation in motion." Especially if you suffer from arthritis, you may soon feel like your old self again!

Take it slow and easy

Here are some tips to keep in mind before you start a tai chi program.

- Wear comfortable shoes and loose clothing.

- A full set of tai chi exercises is called a form. The basic short form has 37 different moves. It can take up to a year to learn the whole form.

- Stay focused on the move you are in and not the one up ahead. Don't move on until you get it right. It's more important to practice tai chi every day than to learn the moves quickly.

- It's extremely important to control your weight shifts. This means when you move, you first shift all your weight onto your supporting leg. Next, place your other foot, and only then move your weight to that leg. This will help you move smoothly. Remember, tai chi should look fluid – not robotic.

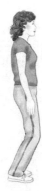

To get into the correct starting position for tai chi, stand with your feet shoulder-width apart, toes pointed forward. Bend your knees just slightly so you drop down about two inches. Don't lean – distribute your weight evenly.

Keep your upper body straight, your head and shoulders relaxed, and your hands loose at your sides. Stand like this for two to three minutes.

Anxious to try out a bit of tai chi? Here are a few moves to whet your appetite.

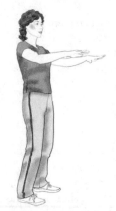 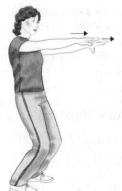 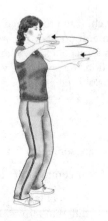

1. Stand with your knees slightly bent. Raise your hands to chest height, palms down, elbows slightly bent.

2. Breathe in.

3. Imagine you're about to swim the breast stroke.

4. Gently extend your arms forward.

5. Sink lower into your knees and breathe out.

6. Keep your back straight, your head up, and your eyes looking forward.

7. Finish the breast-stroke movement by drawing your arms back, in a flat, outward circle. Breathe in.

8. At the same time, straighten slightly to your previous position.

9. Repeat 10 to 30 times.

TAI CHI **Working the oar**

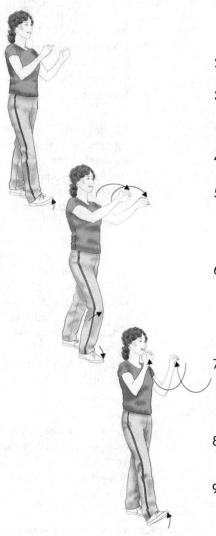

1. Start with your feet about shoulder-width apart. Shift your weight to your left leg.

2. Move your right foot about a foot forward.

3. Raise your hands to chest height, elbows down, and pretend you are holding oars in your hands.

4. Breathe in.

5. Smoothly shift your weight completely onto your right leg. Keep your knee behind the line of your toes.

6. As you breathe out, extend your arms in a forward and downward circular motion, as though rowing.

7. Shift your weight gradually back onto your left foot, lifting the front of your right foot off the floor. Breathe in.

8. Bring your hands back toward your chest to your starting position.

9. Practice this move about 30 times with the right foot forward, then 30 times with the left.

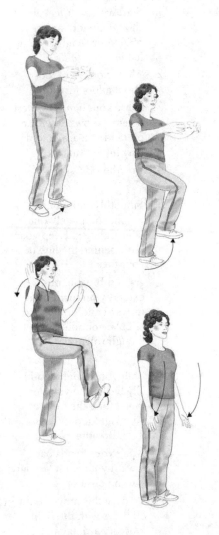

1. From the starting position, shift your weight onto your left foot.
2. Lift your hands to chest height as though you were holding a large balloon.
3. Breathe in.

4. Carefully raise your right leg until your knee is parallel to your hips.
   If you think you might fall over, keep a chair close by. Just don't rest your weight on it.

5. Turn your palms outward. Extend your right foot forward slightly and tilt the sole of your foot out, as though pushing against a wall.
6. Breathe out and hold for 1 second.

7. Lower your foot and bring your arms down to your sides.
8. Repeat 10 to 30 times, alternating feet.

You may see tai chi practiced on beaches and in parks in your area. Join in if you're comfortable with the whole form.

Tai chi offers physical and mental challenges

When Nancy and her husband retired, they needed to burn some energy. Vaguely familiar with tai chi from their years in the Orient, they enrolled in a class together. Both attend once a week and practice three or four times a week at home. They find the new sport surprisingly challenging.

"Like most 'inner arts,' there is much more to tai chi than meets the eye," Nancy says. Had she realized the complexity of it, she would have tried it sooner.

"Tai chi is beneficial on many levels," she explains. "Physically, you must use the strength of your lower body to support your fluid movement. Then, you must work on your balance whenever you step or kick. At the same time, your upper body flexibility is improved by just doing the smooth even movements. Overall coordination is improved just by trying to get upper body movements synchronized with lower body movements."

Nancy emphasizes that tai chi is more than just a physical challenge, however. "It is an excellent mental exercise – learning the order of the form, remembering what direction you should be facing at all times, where your weight is, and where you are going next."

Finally, the deliberate motions and intense focus help her relax. "Tai chi is calming. You must be present in the moment and leave your other worries or life concerns behind."

After almost a year of practice, Nancy finds tai chi deeply gratifying. "It is an art or discipline I can carry with me and can practice in a rather small space. It requires no special clothing or equipment, and it can be satisfying no matter how much or how little time I have available."

Stretch and strengthen with Pilates

In the early 1900s, Joseph Pilates developed a new form of physical therapy that combined Eastern and Western ideas about fitness.

Borrowing from yoga and the gymnastics of ancient Greek and Roman regimens, it focuses on stretching and lengthening the muscles, and improving posture. At the core of his program are six principles: breath, concentration, control, centering, precision, and flow.

Strict Pilates is a combination of mat work and machine-aided exercises. The mat work is easy to learn and can be practiced anywhere. The movements are slow, graceful, and best of all – low-impact. They are so effective, you can forget traditional sit-ups! These exercises will even flatten a bulging belly and strengthen your back, while improving your posture and balance.

Of the three movement therapies, Pilates is the most physically demanding, vigorous enough to qualify as a strength-training program. But you will see speedy results – many people notice a difference after just 10 to 20 sessions. When combined with a cardiovascular exercise, like walking or swimming, Pilates is a full-body fitness program.

Get flatter abs

■ As the name suggests, all you need for the Pilates mat work is a good exercise mat and comfortable clothing. Socks or bare feet work best.

■ Keep your tummy tucked in while doing Pilates moves. Draw the muscles in your abdomen toward your spine, sort of like pulling in to zip up tight pants. If you tighten your lower back and buttocks muscles at the same time, it's called "engaging your powerhouse."

■ For the correct stance – called "foot position" – stand with your feet in a "V" shape, heels together and toes slightly open. Squeeze your buttocks and thighs together. This will twist your calves out slightly. The position is actually the same even if you're lying down and your feet are in the air.

■ When you're told to lift your head off the mat, keep a bit of space between your chin and chest, and always look straight ahead. If this is difficult, you can leave your head down, or prop it on a towel or cushion.

- Don't hold your breath during any exercise. Keep breathing deeply the entire time – in through the nose and out through the mouth.

- Concentrate fully on each motion – focus on your body, on lengthening the muscles and maintaining good posture.

- Not sure about the moves? Consider a session with a trained Pilates instructor. She can explain the machines, and make sure you're using proper form so you don't get hurt.

Time to get started! Here are five exercises to help you banish an unsightly belly, and give you leaner abdominal muscles.

PILATES **The hundred**

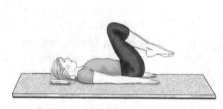

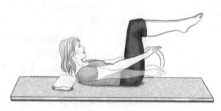

1. Lie on your back and draw your knees in toward your chest.
   Make sure your entire spine touches the mat.

2. Engage your power-house and bring your head and shoulders up.

3. Lift your feet up so your toes are just above knee level.

4. Lift your arms until they are parallel with the floor.

5. Pump your arms up and down, keeping them straight and stretched.
   Pump 5 times while you breathe in, and 5 times as you breathe out.

6. See if you can make it to 50 pumps without stopping. Eventually you should work up to 100 pumps.

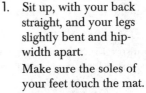

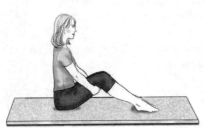

1. Sit up, with your back straight, and your legs slightly bent and hip-width apart.
   Make sure the soles of your feet touch the mat.

2. Wrap your hands under your thighs, close to your knees. Keep your shoulders down and your elbows pointed out like wings.

3. Tighten your buttocks and curve in your abdomen. Slowly lower your back down to the mat.

4. Imagine curling one vertebra down at a time. Keep your back and buttocks in a soft "c" curve.

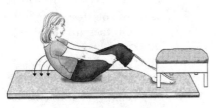

5. As you roll, tuck your chin down and look at your abdomen.

6. Roll down as far as you can without letting go of your thighs. You may want to tuck your feet under a stool.

7. Hold for 3 deep breaths, then lift up gradually until you are back in a seated position.

8. Repeat 3 times.

PILATES **Single leg stretch**

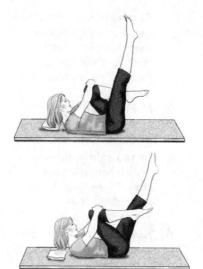

1. Lie on your back, with both knees pulled up to your chest.
2. Lift up and, with both hands, gently hug your left knee toward your shoulder. Keep your elbows pointed out like wings.
3. Point your right leg toward the ceiling.

4. Smoothly switch legs and repeat on the other side. Make sure your hips don't swivel but stay firmly against the mat.
5. Repeat 5 to 8 times.

PILATES **Single leg circle**

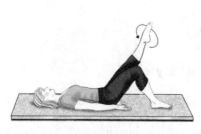

1. Lie flat on your mat, with your arms pressed down at your sides.
2. Bend one knee and point your other leg up at the ceiling.
3. Use your leg like a paintbrush. Pretend to paint circles on the ceiling.
4. Make sure your active hip stays firmly against the mat.
5. Circle 5 times clockwise, then 5 times counter-clockwise. Switch legs and repeat.

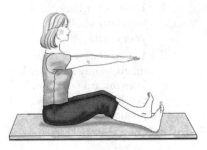

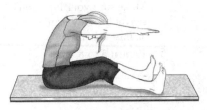

1. Sit straight and tall, with your legs softly bent and about hip-width apart. Point your toes up, as if your feet are pushing against a wall.

2. Hold your arms out straight in front of you at shoulder height.

3. As you exhale, pretend to dive between your arms. Lower your head, and tighten your stomach muscles.

4. Keep your lower back stationary and round your upper back.

5. Stretch forward, as if trying to reach the far wall.

6. Uncurl as you inhale, returning to your original upright position.

7. Repeat 3 to 5 times.

Find a class that suits your style

These exercise examples are only a taste of what you can discover through professional instruction in yoga, tai chi, or Pilates. If you're considering a class, here are some things to think about first.

■ Many gyms, community centers, local YMCA branches, and even churches and synagogues offer movement therapy workshops. Just make sure your instructor has proper training.

- To find an accredited instructor near you, call one of the following organizations, or catch them on the Internet.

  Yoga Alliance
  877-964-2255
  www.yogaalliance.org

  Taoist Tai Chi Society
  www.taoist.org

  Pilates Method Alliance
  866-573-4945
  www.pilatesmethodalliance.org

- Look into local park or community happenings. Unstructured tai chi groups often meet early in the morning in parks. You shouldn't go here to necessarily learn the tai chi form, but to meet others and to practice and refine your technique.

- If you are uncomfortable with Eastern philosophy, look for a trainer who stresses the physical and not the spiritual benefits of these programs.

- If you can't take a class, check your local library or bookstore for books and videos that can help you learn at home.

Power up to slim down

11

Out-muscle age and weakness

You don't have to be Charles Atlas to power up with strength training. This kind of exercise is a key to fitness for everyone – especially seniors. Stacks of scientific studies prove this. In fact, senior muscles may benefit *more* from strength training than young ones.

Strength training has many names. Resistance training, weight lifting, working out, and pumping iron are just a few. Whatever you call it, it's more valuable, easy, and fun than you probably imagined. For instance, you may not know that strength training can rev up your metabolism and help you burn off more calories around the clock.

It gets results by "stressing" your muscles more than your humdrum daily activities do. This stress could come from doing pushups, pressing a dumbbell above your head, or curling a coffee can. Believe it or not, muscles live for this extra work. It makes them stronger and healthier.

Put the brakes on aging

You lose as much as 40 percent of your muscle strength during your adult life, health experts say. This process – called sarcopenia – starts in your 40s and 50s, when your muscle fibers begin to shrink, become less efficient, and disappear altogether. Sarcopenia leads to the weakness, poor coordination, and bad balance that many seniors suffer.

Strength training halts this process and may even reverse it. According to the latest research, your strength could jump by an amazing 100 percent if you're a weight-lifting senior. Pumping iron works because it encourages your muscles to grow and become more responsive and powerful.

Lifting weights can also build up your bones. When muscles flex during strength training, the bones around them respond like plants to sunlight – they grow.

"Resistance training helps maintain bone density at any age," says Elise White, MPT, a physical therapist. "It doesn't take much. Just a little stress on the bones to mitigate the bone loss that is inevitable as we age."

And it doesn't matter how old you are when you start. "Even seniors with osteoporosis can benefit from low-weight, high-rep resistance training," says White. "It's never too late to start preventing bone loss."

Stronger muscles and bones could help you preserve your freedom and your ability to take care of yourself. After all, you need muscles to walk up stairs and climb out of bed, not to mention carry your groceries and pick up your grandchildren.

Don't fret if you gain weight at first from strength training. Your new muscles weigh more than your old fat. Muscle will burn more calories in the long run.

When you follow a regular lifting program, you'll start seeing muscles you haven't seen since you were 30 years old. Strength training carves muscles until they become lean and well-defined.

And unlike fat, muscles do more than take up space. They're constantly eating up calories – three times as many as fat. They keep churning even when you're not exercising. Don't stop working out for long, though. The more you strength train, the more muscles you'll build, which will help your body burn fat faster. So add some muscle and watch the fat melt away.

Strength training could also add 20 yards to your golf drive, or some extra "umph" to your tennis serve. It may take you to a higher level in whatever sport you're active in. Moreover, extra muscle helps protect your joints and lower back during cardiovascular exercises such as jogging and bicycling.

Get the 'thumbs up' from your doctor

You don't need to play golf or jog, however, to enjoy the power-packed benefits of strength training. Any senior can improve his life with this type of workout. Still, you need to take one important precaution before hitting the weight room.

"Everyone should ideally check with their doctor before beginning any exercise program," advises White. Your doctor will help design a weight-lifting program to suit your health and lifestyle needs. Or he can possibly recommend a fitness specialist to do it. This is particularly important if you smoke, have never exercised before, or have a serious health condition, including:

- osteoporosis

- heart disease

- arthritis

- asthma

- cancer

- recent surgery

- high blood pressure

- orthopedic or other injuries

- chronic joint or back problems

Once you get your doctor's green light, strength training may help you overcome these conditions. Studies show it may ease the pain of arthritis while strengthening bones and joints. It could also heal your heart disease by lowering your blood fat and blood pressure levels. And weight lifting even seems to promote a healthy gastrointestinal system as well as end back pain.

Deal a blow against diabetes

Surprisingly, you may enjoy some of the most dramatic benefits from strength training if you're a type 2 diabetic. It could help you get a grip on glucose control, according to an Australian study of overweight diabetic seniors ages 60 to 80.

In this study, one group of men and women lifted weights three days a week for six months while eating a healthy, low-calorie diet. Another group ate the wholesome diet and did stretching exercises. Both groups lost weight at the end of the research, but only the strength-training seniors gained lean body mass and significantly improved their blood-sugar control.

The scientists Down Under were not sure exactly how it worked. They suspected muscle works like a blood-sugar sponge, absorbing glucose out of your system. The strength-training group gained muscle mass as their blood sugar dropped. The second group, on the other hand, lost some of their muscle mass. So this theory seems to make sense.

As all diabetics know, better blood sugar control means less side effects, like heart disease, nerve and kidney problems, and blindness. You don't need more reasons than these to start pumping iron. But remember – check with your doctor before you head for the gym.

Prepare for a positive experience

You have covered all the bases with your doctor, but that does not mean you can jump right into an exercise routine. The more planning you put into it, the more likely you will stick with it. So take the first step toward a successful program, and decide when and where to work out.

Home or gym – the choice is yours

Hone your muscles at home. You don't have to sweat it out in a crowded, costly gym to get a good workout. It's easy to get a great workout and stay in shape in the privacy of your own home – without spending a dime. Many strength exercises can be done with everyday household items – or with no special equipment at all.

Even if you purchase home gym equipment, you may not have to spend a lot. Consider it a one-time investment that will pay dividends every time you use it. Ask your doctor or the salesperson at a sporting goods store what kind of equipment to buy.

Besides, unlike a gym, your "spa" will always be as clean and quiet as you want it to be. You won't have to compete with other people to use equipment. And, of course, you won't have to travel very far to get to it.

Get slim at the gym. For many people, a gym or health club membership is well worth it. As personal trainer Greg Warner puts it, "The gym has more equipment. Few people have in their home what is in a gym." Gyms also hire trainers like Warner to show you how to use all these fancy machines. "Plus," Warner adds, "it's easier to become motivated when everyone else is working out." On top of all this, gyms are a great place to meet people.

Shop around for a gym if you're interested. Most places offer free passes to let you get the feel of their gym. Find one you're comfortable in, so you'll continue to come back. Try out the national chains – like Bally or Atlas – since they may have several convenient locations in your town. And test the waters at your local YMCA, community center, or church as well.

Seize the best time for a workout

Once you figure out where to strength train, decide when you'll do it. Your best bet, say fitness gurus, is to try for three times a week. Believe it or not, the reason for this may be the rest it allows you. It's important to take at least one day off between sessions. Your muscles need that long to recuperate and grow.

Working your muscles Monday, Wednesday, and Friday will fulfill these requirements. On your off days, you can walk, garden, golf, or do other fitness activities.

Some experts think your muscles are stronger in the afternoon because your body is warmed up. Others say men should exercise in the morning, when their muscle-building hormones peak. Unless you're competing for the next Mr. Universe, however, don't let science tell you when to lift. Pick the time of day that's most convenient for you, and you're more likely to get it done.

If you're an early riser, first thing in the morning may be best. On the other hand, you could try making your lunch

> ### Will strength training bulk up a woman like a man?
>
> No. In general, women don't become muscle-bound from lifting weights. It's just not in most women's genes to go from being Jane to looking like Tarzan.
>
> A study in the *Journal of the American Medical Association* found that women ended up smaller, not larger, after lifting weights. Although their muscles increased an average of 9 percent, they also lost fat. Since muscle is denser, they looked trimmer.
>
> Although women bodybuilders can develop powerful-looking builds, normal strength training will simply make you look leaner, healthier, and more fit.

break more about burning calories than eating them. Or sneak in exercise after work and before dinner. If you go to a gym, the best time may be when the gym is the least busy. Stay flexible, and you'll always fit it in.

Fit in by learning the lingo

To get a grip on working out, it's best to be familiar with some strength-training slang.

- **Exercise.** Each strength-training activity, such as pushups or squats, is called an exercise.

- **Rep.** Short for repetition, this term stands for each time you carry out the motions of an exercise. Doing 15 pushups, for instance, would be doing 15 reps.

- **Set.** A group of reps makes a set. Those 15 pushups would make up your first set, or round, of exercises. If you rested and then did 15 more, that would be your second set.

- **Machines.** These are special lifting devices you find at gyms. You use different machines to work different muscles, although some machines may work more than one muscle group.

- **Barbell.** You can slide weighted metal plates onto this metal bar, which is usually 4 to 6 feet long. That way, you can make a barbell as heavy or as light as you want.

- **Dumbbells.** These are smaller versions of barbells. You use one for each hand.

- **Free weights.** This refers to exercises done with barbells and dumbbells, as well as the barbells and dumbbells themselves.

- **Weight.** This is a generic word for a dumbbell or barbell and the term for the number of pounds it weighs.

- **Bench.** You sit or lie on these padded seats while doing exercises.

Comfort tops the training list

It's important to feel comfortable when you train. Wear loose-fitting clothes, which won't be too hot or too tight. Your typical sweatpants and T-shirt will do the trick. For footwear, try any pair of supportive athletic shoes, including walking shoes, sneakers, or tennis shoes.

Water is also essential to perform at your peak. Drink a glass before you exercise, and sip some throughout your workout. Sports drinks are fine, too, if you prefer a little flavor. Try for six to eight glasses of fluid during the rest of the day. As for food, it's important to eat before a workout, but not *right* before a workout. If your stomach is full, you may not have the energy for lifting weights because your body is busy digesting your food. Exercising on an empty stomach is also a bad idea because you could get lightheaded. Your safe bet is to wait an hour or two after a meal so you can stomach your routine.

Master the rules to achieve your goals

Every strength training exercise has its own stance and movements, which you'll learn in a little bit. But before you grasp those, it's important to first master these universal rules. They can help you prevent injury no matter which exercise you're doing.

Practice good posture. Always stand or sit straight. Keep your chin in and lined up with your neck and back. Unlock your knees and leave them flexible. If you're seated, angle your knees at 90 degrees.

Relax. Let your body be loose. Allow your shoulders to hang in their natural position. Tense only the particular muscle you're exercising at the time.

Posture is important when picking up weights from a rack or off the ground. Always let your legs do the work — not your back.

Slow down. Whether the exercise calls for you to push or pull, move the weights and your muscles slowly. As a rough guide, take two to three seconds to do an exercise's flexing motion. Hold it for a second. Then spend four to five seconds returning to the starting position.

Concentrate. Never jerk, swing, or bounce a dumbbell or barbell. That's one way injuries occur. Always have control over the weight, and stay within a comfortable range of motion. If you can't, you may be tired. Stop and rest for the next set.

Breathe. Sounds simple enough, but if you don't breathe while you work out, your blood pressure could shoot through the roof. Most experts recommend exhaling while you contract your muscle and inhaling when you relax. But don't think too hard about it – just breathe like you normally would.

Take a day off. Listen to your body. Pass on exercise when you feel under-the-weather, tired, or overly sore. Working out then may only make you feel worse.

Keep pain in check

Experts say you don't need to strain or feel pain to get stronger and more fit. Still, you will feel *something* if you strength train correctly. Just be sure it's a healthy feeling in your muscles and not a danger sign. Here's what to look for:

- **"Good" pain.** This warmth and tightness happens naturally any time you use a muscle repeatedly. Afterward, you may ache all over, especially if you haven't lifted weights before. Once your muscles get used to the activity, you'll feel this soreness less and less.

- **"Bad" pain.** If you feel sharp pains in your bones or joints while you exercise, that's not natural. Stop exercising immediately, and notify your trainer. You may need to see your doctor.

If you have a serious health condition, strength training can bring on other "bad" pains, too, like chest pain or pressure, breathing trouble, lightheadedness, dizziness, nausea, and even unconsciousness. If you feel any of these, stop exercising. Notify your doctor immediately.

Get pumped for the new you

It's time to fashion your own strength-training workout. In the following pages, you'll find exercises that pump up your muscles from head to toe. They include step-by-step directions and illustrations showing you how to perform each exercise properly. To arrange these exercises into a valuable and fun routine, follow these time-tested guidelines.

- Warm up before each and every training session. "Five to 10 minutes of light cardio will help increase the blood flow to the muscles, ensuring you get maximum benefit out of the strength training, and will help prevent injury," explains White. A brisk walk to the gym, calisthenics, or even washing your car would count.

- Make your workout complete by exercising all six major muscle groups – chest, back, legs, arms, shoulders, and abdominals (abs). This guarantees you'll hit complementary, or opposite, muscles, such as the muscles on the front and back of your arms (biceps and triceps) and the front and back of your legs (quadriceps and hamstrings). By exercising these pairs, you'll build a balanced, flexible, and injury-free body.

- Schedule the biggest muscle groups – chest, back, and legs – in your workout before the smaller ones – shoulders, arms, and abs. Bigger muscles take more energy to exercise, so you'll need to be fresh to do your best.

- Pick one to two exercises for every muscle group.

- Do one set of 10 to 15 reps for each exercise.

- Rest two to three minutes in between each set.

- Add another five minutes at the end of your workout for relaxing cool-down stretches.

- Expect this workout to take at least 20 minutes and no more than 45 minutes at a slow, controlled pace.

- Spend your first workout getting accustomed to the exercises. Warner's advice to his clients? "I tell them not to overexert themselves on the first day. We err on the side of safety at light, comfortable weights. Form is emphasized." So get a feel for technique and posture before pushing yourself.

Once you get the hang of it, determine how many pounds you should lift for each exercise. "It's almost trial by error," Warner explains. "Again, you should start very light and gradually work your way up."

For the best workout, use the heaviest weight you can lift for at least 10 but no more than 15 repetitions. You may want to ask a trainer for help if you're working out in a gym.

Keep track of your workouts with a small notebook and pen. At every session, write down the exercises you did, the amount of weight used, and the number of reps.

Once you figure out what works best for each exercise, stick with those weights for your first few workouts, then raise them as you progress to the next level.

Set higher goals for top results

It may only take a few sessions to see amazing results from strength training. The first sign may be no soreness the day after a workout. Next, you could notice how energized you feel all day long. Then your workouts may become easier and easier.

There must be a catch to all of these benefits, you say? Actually, there is. Your muscles will get accustomed to your workout, and your progress will slow down. This occurs because of what health experts call the "overload principle." It's a fancy way to say your muscles like to always be tested. They don't get a kick from doing the same exercise routine over and over. To give your muscles a run for their money and guarantee results, change your workout often. Here's how.

Steel your muscles with more sets. "Increase the number of reps per set, and the number of sets per session," White recommends. Raising your reps to 15 is your best bet, according to most experts. Then when that gets to be a breeze, complete two sets of the exercise instead of just one. Advance to three sets if you can handle it.

Wield more weight. "When that becomes easy," White says, "then increase the weight." Warner agrees. "Depending upon your goals," he says, "one usually should increase weight when they can perform 15 reps with ease."

Many exercises require only an investment of time — not money. Some need no equipment at all. For exercises that need weights, substitute soup cans or any graspable household item.

A safe increase is 10 percent of your previous weight. So, for instance, if you were doing military presses with 20 pounds, raise your weight to 22 pounds (or the closest dumbbell available).

Rotate your exercises. "If the routine gets too easy or boring," White continues, "try adding new exercises for each body part." In other words, swap exercises. Instead of lateral dumbbell raises, for instance, switch to front dumbbell raises for your shoulders. For legs, try lunges instead of squats. This will shock your muscles, as well as jumpstart your enthusiasm.

Recruit a friend. "Also," Warner suggests, "working out with someone will push you to work harder." So find a friend who is interested in getting fit. You'll encourage each other and keep one another company.

Transform your workout. If you really enjoy strength training but your workout isn't tough enough, try a radical change. Serious body builders use many different workout arrangements to motivate their muscles. Talk with a physical trainer about these other workout possibilities.

Turn it up with a trainer. You still may benefit from talking with a trainer even if you don't want a major overhaul in your workout schedule. A trainer is an expert in helping people realize their fitness goals. "If everything seems to be going well but you're just not seeing the results you want," White advises, "a trainer has a plethora of different exercises to keep things from getting boring and help move you along."

Easy exercises to power up

Now that you understand the basics, here are the exercises you need to put them into motion. By no means are these the only exercises out there. But these are all great for beginning lifters, not to mention easy ways to boost your metabolism and burn fat. The no-sweat back workout will also build up your back and help banish your back pain. Once you learn what muscles to strengthen to make your back feel better, you may no longer have to live with chronic pain. Try these and the other weight-bearing exercises, and watch how quickly your body will tone up and become stronger.

CHEST Wall press

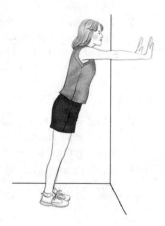

1. Stand facing a wall at arms' length.
2. Place both of your hands against the wall at shoulder height.

CHEST **Wall press**

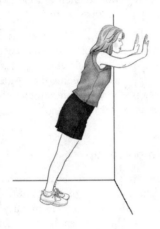

3. Bend your elbows, and slowly lower your chest toward the wall.
4. Push yourself back up to finish the rep.

CHEST **Modified knee push-up**

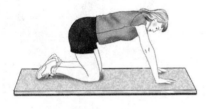

1. Get down on your hands and knees.
2. Lay your hands on the floor below but slightly ahead of your shoulders.

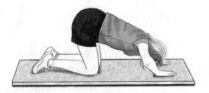

3. Bend your elbows, and lower your chest as close to the ground as possible.
4. Push yourself back up to end the rep.

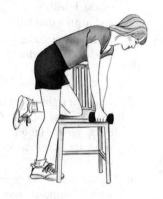

1. Stand to the right of a chair or flat bench. Place a dumbbell on the floor to the chair's right.

2. Rest your left knee on the chair, lean forward, and plant your left hand on the chair. Grab the dumbbell with your right hand.

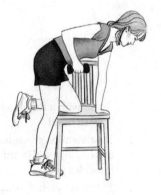

3. Keeping your back parallel to the chair, pull the weight up toward your chest.

4. Lower the weight to end the rep. After 10 to 15 reps, switch and work your left arm.

BACK **Back extension**

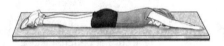

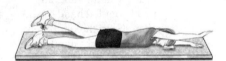

1. Lie face down on your stomach with your legs and arms extended.
2. Fold a towel under your forehead for padding.

3. Lift your right arm and left leg a few inches off the ground. Tighten your stomach muscles while lifting.
4. Lower them, and repeat with the opposite arm and leg to finish the rep.

BACK/SHOULDERS **Shoulder shrug**

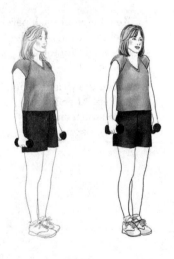

1. Stand with a dumbbell in each hand.
2. Rest them on the sides of your legs with your knuckles out.
3. Pull your shoulders up toward your ears, leaving your arms straight.
4. Lower them back down to end the rep.

BACK/SHOULDERS **Upward row**

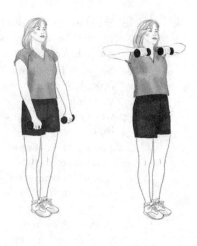

1. Stand holding a dumb-bell in each hand.
2. Let your arms hang down with the weights in front of your body and your knuckles out.
3. Move the weights toward your chin by pulling your hands straight up.
4. Stop at shoulder height, and lower the weights back down to finish the rep.

LEGS **No-weight squat**

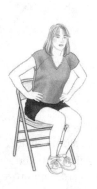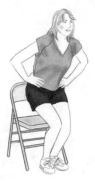

1. Sit on a sturdy chair or flat bench.
2. Hold your hands on your hips for balance.
3. Lean forward and stand up, keeping your body centered over your feet.
4. Sit back down to end the rep.

LEGS **Lunge**

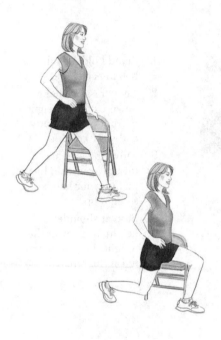

1. Stand to the right of a sturdy chair, which you can hold for support.
2. Set your feet about three feet apart, with your left foot forward and your right foot in back.
3. Bend both knees and lower your body straight down. Don't allow your front knee to go past your toe.
4. Push back up and stand to end the rep. After 10 to 15 reps, switch leg positions and repeat.

LEGS **Back leg swing**

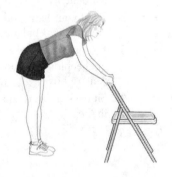

1. Stand one to two feet behind a sturdy chair.
2. Bend at the waist and lean forward, supporting yourself on the back of the chair.

LEGS Back leg swing

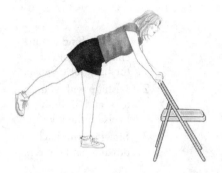

3. Raise your right leg straight behind you until it's in line with your back.
4. Return your foot to the floor to end the rep. After 10 to 15 reps with your right leg, switch to your left.

LEGS Side leg swing

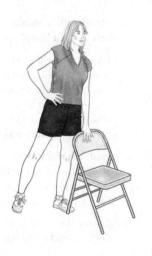

1. Stand behind a sturdy chair, and hold the back for balance.
2. Slowly lift your right leg straight out to the side until it's 6 inches off the ground.
3. Lower your foot to the floor to end the rep. After 10 to 15 reps, switch to your left leg and repeat.

LEGS **Calf raise**

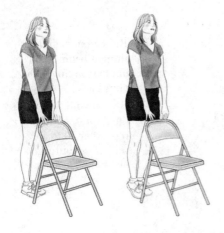

1. Stand behind a sturdy chair, and hold on to the back for balance.
2. Push up with your toes, and lift both heels off the floor.
3. Slowly lower back down to end the rep.

SHOULDERS **Military press**

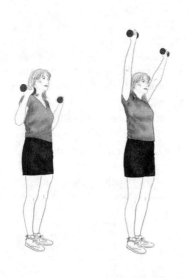

1. Stand with a dumb-bell in each hand.

2. Raise the weights to your shoulders. Keep your arms below your shoulders with your elbows bent and your palms facing forward.

3. Push the dumbbells above your head until your arms are straight. Don't arch your back.

4. Lower the weights to your shoulders to end the rep.

SHOULDERS Lateral dumbbell raise

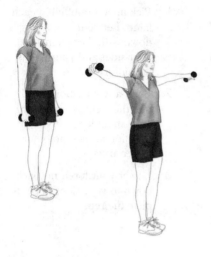

1. Stand with a dumb-bell in each hand.
2. Rest them on the sides of your hips with your knuckles out.
3. Slowly raise your arms out to the sides, keeping your elbows slightly bent.
4. Stop at shoulder height, and lower them back down to finish the rep.

SHOULDERS Front dumbbell raise

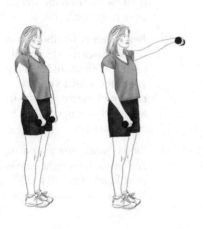

1. Stand with a dumb-bell in each hand.
2. Rest them on the front of your thighs with your knuckles out.
3. Slowly raise your left arm in front of you, keeping your elbows slightly bent.
4. Stop at shoulder height, and lower it back down. Raise and lower your right arm to end the rep.

ARMS **Bicep curl**

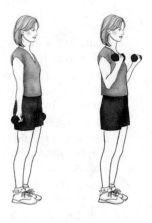

1. Pick up a dumbbell in each hand. Let your arms hang down with the weights at your sides and your palms facing forward.

2. Bend at your elbows, and pull the weights up toward your shoulders. Move only your forearms – not your upper arms.

3. Lower your forearms back down to your sides to complete the rep.

ARMS **Overhead tricep extension**

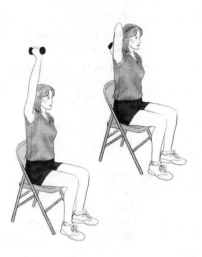

1. Sit with a dumbbell in your right hand. Hold the weight over your head.

2. Bend your right elbow, and slowly lower the dumbbell toward your shoulder. Keep your elbow near your ear, pointing forward. Use your left hand to support your arm, if needed.

3. Slowly straighten your arm, and press the weight above your head. After 10 to 15 reps, switch arms and repeat.

ARMS Tricep kickback

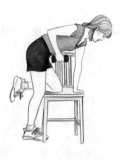

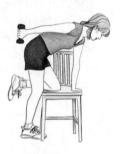

1. Place a dumbbell on a chair or flat bench. Standing to the right of the chair, rest your left knee on it and lean forward over the weight.
2. Place your left hand on the bench. Pick up the dumbbell with your right hand. Cock your elbow back so your arm makes an L. Keep your back straight.
3. Straighten your right arm, pushing the weight backward. Only your forearm should move – not your whole arm.
4. Lower your forearm back into the L position to finish the rep. After 10 to 15 reps with your right arm, repeat with your left.

ABS Abdominal press

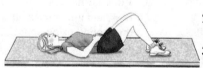

1. Lie on the floor or bed on your back.
2. Bend your knees, and plant your feet on the floor.
3. Flatten the small of your back against the floor using your stomach muscles.
4. Hold. Relax to end the rep.

ABS Leg lift

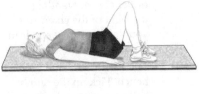

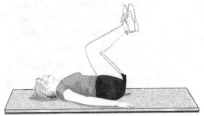

1. Lie on the floor on your back. Bend your knees, and plant your feet on the floor a foot or two from your buttocks.
2. Lift your legs off the ground, and bring your thighs as close to your ribs as possible. Squeeze your abdominals.
3. Lower your legs so they almost touch the ground to complete one rep.

ABS Crunch

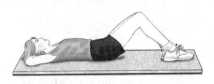

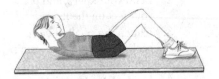

1. Lie on the floor on your back. Fold your hands behind your head.
2. Bend your knees, and plant your feet on the floor about a foot from your buttocks.
3. Lift your head, shoulders, and upper back off the ground using your stomach muscles – not your arms.
4. Lower yourself to the ground to end the rep.

Turn back the years with strength training

If all this talk about bending and lifting makes you wonder if strength training is for you, just listen to 70-year-old Yvette Boucher.

"Before I moved here to Florida," she recalls, "the doctor said I would be in a wheelchair in about five years. That was 12 years ago."

You may think it was the Southern sun that helped Yvette overcome her crippling arthritis. But she thanks strength training. It's what powers her busy lifestyle.

"What I like the most," she confides, "is that it gives me the energy to do whatever I want the rest of the day, and it makes you look and feel a lot younger than most people I know my age who don't exercise."

Listen to this on-the-go senior's exercise schedule, and you'll be even more impressed.

"I still play golf twice a week, and I try to keep as active as possible," Yvette says. "I do a little of everything, starting with the upper body one day, aerobics the second day, and the lower body the third. I go six times a week for one hour a day."

"I started this strength training program from the advice of my daughter who is a physical therapist," she explains. "Best advice she ever gave me."

So follow Yvette's advice. You don't have to match her workout. Start with as much exercise as you feel comfortable with. Strength training is not about lifting the heaviest weight or getting the biggest biceps. It's about having fun while staying fit.

"I guarantee you, too, will feel better," Yvette assures, "and you will be motivated to keep on as long as you can."

Making fitness fun 12

Turn a good workout into a good time

Are you having fun yet? If you look forward to your fitness activities, you're more likely to stick with them. If you're not enjoying getting fit, it's not too late. You can still whittle the work out of your workout and make exercise more exhilarating.

To bring some zing to your fitness plan, start by tweaking your activities just a little, then consider more dramatic changes. To breathe new life into an old fitness plan, try the ideas in this chapter – and see how much more fun fitness can be.

Change your routine

If you're in a fitness rut, see if these ideas can work for you.

- Try a new time. If you work out in the morning, road test a switch to later in the day. Have you been exercising in the evening when you're already tired? Perhaps a morning workout would be better.

- Shift your schedule. Are all your fitness activities done on weekdays? Try planning some for the weekend.

- Take the inside out – or bring the outside in. A taste of sunlight and fresh air might be just the thing to revitalize you. On the other hand, an indoor routine may be a welcome change on certain days.

- Head for a new location. Try to think of a place that's scenic, interesting, or distracting in some way and take your exercise there. Ride your bike through a different subdivision or play tennis at a new court. Walk in a mall, a local park, or even an inexpensive zoo.

- Mix it up. If you walk, jog, or bike along a specific route, consider trying that path in reverse – even if you only use a fitness track. Is your workout a series of exercises? Find out if you can safely perform them in a different order. This may work well for calisthenics, strength exercises, or even stretches.

- Join the crowd. Check out a club or a league dedicated to your favorite sport. Both can be great places to exchange tips and tricks while enjoying your favorite pastime. You can even find senior leagues or over-50 leagues exclusively for older adults. These leagues exist for baseball, softball, hockey, basketball, soccer, and more.

Take the "class-y" approach

For all out boredom-busting, take a class in a sport or exercise you've never tried before. You're less likely to lose interest when you're learning something new at every class. You can get pointers from others and, perhaps, make new friends.

Or sign up for a refresher course in your exercise of choice and you can check your technique, make adjustments, and get more satisfying results. Watch carefully and ask questions to get the full advantage of your instructor's expertise and experience.

To find classes, check the YMCA or YWCA, senior centers, churches, hospitals, colleges or universities, wellness centers, health clubs, and your city, state, or regional office on aging.

Exercise videos can be your class away from class. Rent or buy a video to sample instructor-guided fitness right in your own home. What's more, you can try classes that may not be available in your area.

Mix fitness with pleasure

Getting fit can even be part of a relaxing vacation, a fun weekend, or a simple day trip. Let these tips get you started.

- Look for a state or national park within easy driving distance and go for a scenic fitness getaway. You can choose how long to stay, how much to spend, and whether to exercise a lot or just a little.

  Take scenic strolls, go bird watching, or even try a short hike. Look for something new like canoeing or horseback riding. How about biking trails or a biking tour? And then there are guided nature walks that may introduce you to anything from wildflowers to caves.

- Scan your local paper for upcoming events. A tour through a large museum or exhibit makes for interesting – and educational – walking. Inexpensive fairs and festivals can be fun walks, too.

- If you're planning a vacation, pack fitness into your trip. Hunt for seashells at the beach. Walk or bike for better sightseeing. In fact, one New York City resident offers this tip for seeing the Big Apple. "On a summer weekend, when traffic is light, biking is a wonderful way to see the city." He recommends it to tourists who want an off-the-beaten-path agenda.

Be a kid again

Becoming more active can be child's play – literally. Even if you're not a kid anymore, childhood games can still help you get fit. Just be sure to check with your doctor before you start.

Play with your kids or grandkids, and you'll blend the fun of a second childhood with healthy exercise. Tag, hide and seek, and kickball are just a few old favorites to try – even if you have to adjust the rules a bit for slower, safer play. Grab your favorite little leaguer for a bit of catch, or go out for a game of miniature golf. You'll get quality family time along with quality fitness time.

Take your dog for a walk every day to keep both of you fit and healthy.

Childhood toys can definitely burn some calories and work some muscles. If your doctor approves, swing a hula-hoop, jump rope, or toss a flying disc – or Frisbee – with a pal.

For extra action, try out disc golf. In this airborne version, you aim your flying disc for a hoop or basket.

Sample something new and exciting

Do you have just one exercise activity you do all the time? Why not spice up the routine by alternating a day of aerobic exercise, for example, with a day of strength training. People who speak athletic lingo call this cross training.

Of course, if your current exercise is totally boring, switch to something altogether different. Your new activity can be a standard exercise – such as calisthenics or strength training – or a new sport.

Hobbies, too, are a fantastic way to sneak fitness into your day. After all, people were strong and fit centuries before gyms, classes, and exercise machines came along. Gardening, dancing, games, sports, and even just getting from one place to another are all good workouts. Consider the following fitness activities. You might find the right one for you.

Harvest good health in your own back yard

A health-building fitness center may be just outside your front door. Whether you dream of a garden lush enough to grace a magazine cover or simply want a neat lawn, you can get great exercise from yard work.

At first glance, it might not seem like a workout, yet when you dig, rake, and plant, you are expending more energy than when you play golf or walk the dog.

The toughest gardening workouts come from specific tasks like mowing the lawn with a push mower, chopping wood, shoveling, or tilling. These activities burn as many calories as doubles tennis, fencing, downhill skiing, and playing softball.

As you can see, gardening burns calories, builds muscle, and even improves flexibility. The following numbers from the Calorie Control Council, a non-profit association representing the low-calorie and reduced-fat food and beverage industry, show how many calories a 150-pound person can burn in just 30 minutes of yard work.

Yard or garden task	Calories burned
Stacking firewood	207
Shoveling snow	203
Raking	171
General gardening	162
Mowing lawn	162

And if that's not enough, spending some time and energy in your garden can do more. Scientific research reports gardening may be one of the best activities for building bones – right up there with lifting weights.

Women who gardened at least once a week had higher bone density than women who did other exercises. In addition, when you're exposed to the sun, your body creates extra bone-boosting vitamin D. So say goodbye to the brittle bones of osteoporosis and hello to a stronger you.

But that's not all. Fresh fruits and vegetables from your garden offer healthy produce for your table.

The aroma of fragrant blossoms or herbs – like lavender – can help drive off the blues.

Got allergies? Avoid gardening before 10 a.m. when pollen counts are highest.

And you'll just feel good about yourself and your accomplishments after creating a beautiful yard or garden.

Even better, gardening can be both convenient and fun. When you garden for fitness, you skip the hassle and cost of going to a gym. Nobody pushes you. You decide how hard and how long to work. In short, gardening is a fun workout you can do on your own terms.

To make gardening work well for you, try these tips.

- Begin your gardening session by warming up, and make sure you cool down slowly afterward.

- Rome wasn't built in a day and your dream yard or garden shouldn't be either. Set small goals. For instance, spend only 20 to 30 minutes weeding or pruning at a time.

- Try switching hands occasionally when raking, hoeing, or digging.

- Use duct tape to attach a broomstick onto your trowel and you'll never have to bend over again. Make sure your fork and spade have handles long enough to reach your waist.

  Keep an eye out for other tools and ideas that could make gardening easier. Check garden supply stores and catalogs for garden tools designed to prevent strain and soreness.

- If you do the same task for long periods, you're more likely to get stiff and sore. Do a few minutes of weeding here and a few minutes of planting there. Never keep at one task for too long.

- Kneepads aren't just for risky sports. Wear them in the garden so you won't have to move a knee cushion every time you reposition.

- Fill an old play wagon with mulch and fertilizer. Stack small items on a skateboard or sled. Pulling and dragging are easier on your back than lifting and carrying.

- Bend at your knees, not at your waist.

- Take frequent breaks to stop and stretch, especially if you spend a lot of time kneeling. Besides, it's the ideal place and time to stop and smell the roses.

Dance for fun and fitness

If a bit of the old soft shoe is not in your current game plan for getting fit, rethink your strategy. Dancing can be a terrific aerobic exercise that improves your flexibility and tones your muscles. It's also a weight-bearing activity – good for anyone concerned about bone loss from osteoporosis.

Anne Green Gilbert, author of *Creative Dance for All Ages* and creator of the *BrainDance* video, explains how dance can help your body. "Most dance styles are based on walking patterns so they all build lower body muscle groups."

But she says you can build upper body strength with dances requiring a partner, like ballroom dance, square dance, jazz dance, folk dance, modern dance, and ballet.

"Dances that include turns and spins, tipping and dipping – anything that takes us off balance – will strengthen the balance system," she adds.

And just because dance can have aerobic benefits, Gilbert says you don't have to wear yourself out. "Any form of dance can be slowed down to make it less demanding."

Dr. Susan Spalding, Director of Dance Programs at Berea College, sums it up nicely. "In general, dance is good for cardiovascular fitness, strength, endurance, and flexibility."

If you'd like to try dance for fitness, ask yourself these questions to help you decide which style of dance to try.

- What kind of music do you enjoy? If you like country songs, zydeco, or bluegrass music, square dancing may be for you. If you love swing, music from past decades, or Latin music, you might try ballroom dance.

■ Would you rather dance alone, with a partner, or as part of a group? Ballroom dance, for instance, requires a partner, but you can participate in any line dance without one.

■ Are classes available in your area, or can you be happy learning from a video? A local hula instructor may be tough to find.

■ What type of dance have you always dreamed of trying? Pick one you're really interested in. If you're motivated by a true love of the dance, you'll be more inclined to stick with it as part of your fitness regimen.

Get fit as a fiddle with square dance

Square dancing and its close cousin contra dance are two festive dances that can be great for fitness. Both are informal group dances led by a caller whose cheerful patter guides you from one dance move to the next.

Square dancing usually starts with four couples arranged in a small square. Once the music begins, the caller prompts the dancers through various movements that feature a smooth, shuffling walk. If you can walk to music, you can learn to square dance, although you may need anywhere from five to nine months of lessons before you feel you can dance just for fun – but even the lessons should be enjoyable.

Contra dancing is a bit different. You don't even need lessons. Dancers begin by facing each other – directly across from a partner – in two long lines. The caller first talks you through the entire dance, then when the music begins, you're ready to go with just a little help from the caller's prompts.

According to Spalding, square dancing is usually a less intense, aerobic workout than contra dancing. "Square dancing is probably closer to walking in terms of impact, and contra dancing is probably closer to step aerobics," she explains. "However, in some communities, people clog while they are doing old time square dancing, and that elevates the heart rate considerably."

Both types of dancing can boost your endurance and strengthen your back and legs while working muscles in your upper arms, stomach, and hips. These dances may also improve the flexibility in the "shoulder girdle" – your collarbone, shoulders, and the area between your shoulder blades. To work toward these benefits, Spalding suggests dancing three times a week.

To find out where to go for lessons or dancing, contact the Folk Dance Association at 1-888-321-1023 or write them at:

P.O. Box 300500
Brooklyn, NY 11230-0500

If you prefer, send an e-mail to: director@folkdancing.org. You can also visit their Web site at <www.folkdancing.org>. If you write or e-mail, be sure to include your name and phone number.

Waltz your way into shape with ballroom dance

Are you a fan of the foxtrot? Are you sold on the samba? Then take a chance on ballroom dance.

It does take two to tango – or participate in any other ballroom dance, for that matter. And that's why ballroom dance is also called social dance. Besides traditional favorites like the waltz and foxtrot, you can learn swing dances, novelty dances, or even Latin dances like the cha cha or rumba.

"Ballroom or Latin dancing is a great workout and a lot of fun for all ages," says professional ballroom dancer and instructor Gillian Grimsley of Atlanta. "I know several students in their 90s still going strong and competing! And they swear that dancing has kept them alive and in such good shape. Even their doctors have told them that."

"I believe that all movement helps keep the brain active."
– Anne Green Gilbert, author, *Creative Dance for All Ages*

As a certified personal trainer and aerobics and Jazzercise instructor, Grimsley knows how ballroom dancing can work muscles and improve fitness.

"All muscle groups will get a good workout with ballroom dances," Grimsley says. "The way you hold your arms up with your partner works the upper back. And the abs (abdominals) always get a good workout because in order to keep a good posture, you must stand up straight at all times and keep your abs pulled in."

Ballroom dance also builds your lower body, as Grimsley explains. "In Latin dances, the hip and waist especially get the most workout. In both ballroom and Latin, you must stay 'grounded' – low to the ground with knees bent – which is a great lower body workout."

"A beginning student," she says, "would see an improvement in both tone and strength after a month or more of classes."

Expect a good aerobic workout from ballroom dance, as well. Grimsley says most are low impact, but advanced swing dance or jive can be a high impact workout for those who want one.

Ballroom dancing is also called DanceSport. The International Olympic Committee recognizes it as a sport and may someday include it in the summer games.

You can also improve balance, flexibility, coordination, and agility while you're having fun dancing. "And," says Grimsley, "the more you dance and the more advanced you become, the more these will improve."

If you want to learn ballroom dance, try the sources listed earlier in this chapter to see if classes are available. You can also request information from the United States Amateur Ballroom Dancers Association (USABDA). Call them at 1-800-447-9047. Or write:

PO Box 128
New Freedom, PA 17349

If you already know how to dance, where can you go to cut a rug? "Most dance studios offer weekly ballroom dances," Grimsley says, "and so do Knights of Columbus locations."

Let line dancing liven up your life

Line dancing isn't just for country music fans anymore. Folks are toe-tapping to all kinds of music as they stand shoulder to shoulder and perform the trademark steps and quarter turns of this fun dance. But can this really be a way to get fit?

"It's an all around good type of exercise," says Cynthia Baldwin, a line dance instructor at Gold's Gym in Georgia. She believes even beginners can look forward to many fitness benefits.

"They'll learn to balance, use rhythm, timing, poise, and posture," Baldwin explains. "And it promotes your cardiovascular health."

Over time, dancers may also see improvements in lower body strength and muscle tone. According to Baldwin, line dancing may even help keep your memory in good working order. After all, when you focus on remembering dance steps, you're exercising your brain as well as your body.

Line dancing is good aerobic exercise, but if you haven't already mastered aerobic fitness, don't worry. You can still take a line dance class like Baldwin's. "We'll start at the beginner level and then we'll work our way up," she promises.

Line dancers are also free to choose how hard to exercise. "If they want to stay on the beginner level, then they do so. If they feel like they're flexible and agile enough to move at a faster speed, then they can – and they can do it at their own pace." When it comes to line dancing, Baldwin says, age is not a factor.

Connecticut resident Tess Pawlak would agree with that. At 79, she's been line dancing for three years and attends four classes a week. "The teacher we have now is about 93," she says. "And that woman is a wonderful dancer."

Before the music begins, they walk through the dance as a class. "The first time you try it, you probably won't learn it all," Tess admits. "But, there are a lot of new people who join, so they have to go over it. And once you keep doing it over and over, you will learn it."

Take her advice and find a spot in the middle of the class or near the front. That way, no matter which way the dance turns, you'll be able to watch and learn from another dancer.

Keep pushing yourself, but don't bite off more than you can chew. According to Tess, a lot of people are out of breath when they first start. "But, when you keep going, it's wonderful. If you don't feel up to it, you just sit down. And then you get up and do it again."

"It's very inexpensive," she adds. "We pay a little fee like $3 or $5 and go to a senior center for about an hour. Sometimes they have what they call record hops. It's something I enjoy doing because I don't have a spouse. You can go and not feel that you have to have a partner with you."

Although there are social benefits, Tess says, "I'm doing it for the exercise. The reason I took up line dancing is because I wanted to get my heart rate up and bring my blood pressure down."

And all that fun has paid off. "My blood pressure and heart rate are stable," she reports. "I've trimmed down a little and I'm a little more flexible. I'm pretty good, according to my doctor."

Tess has also found two ways that line dance classes can remove barriers to getting fit.

■ Bad weather can curb anyone's enthusiasm for outdoor workouts. "I don't like to walk in the cold," Tess says. Instead, she enjoys line dancing indoors year round.

■ A dance class can keep you committed to fitness. When you know other people are expecting you to be at class at a certain time, you're more likely to go – and less likely to postpone a workout.

"It's friendly and it's social," Baldwin says of line dancing. "People can get away from the stress going on in the world today. The whole family can do it, in fact."

Line dancing classes are getting easier to find. Check for them wherever you find general dance or exercise classes.

Bring your fitness up to par

Would you rather swing a golf club than swing your partner? Then perhaps golf is your course to fitness.

Golf is an outdoor game. Your goal is to use a club to send a small ball into each distant hole – preferably in as few swings as possible. No two golf courses are the same, so each one is a fresh challenge.

If you're new to the game, take lessons. They should help you learn how to pick the right club, perfect your swing, and guide your ball through such tricky terrain as high grass, sand traps, water hazards, and hills.

> **For bargains on golf clubs, tennis rackets, and other sports items, try second-hand sports equipment stores or yard and garage sales.**

Be sure to plan for several expenses – you'll need clubs, golf balls, and greens fees.

The American Heart Association says golf is a good low-intensity exercise for older adults. If you're up to golfing without a cart, you may reap extra benefits. In just 20 weeks, middle-aged golfers who played cart-free about twice a week reduced their waistline, increased their HDL (good) cholesterol, and lost weight.

The study also suggests that playing golf regularly — without a cart — can strengthen your mid-body muscles and so reduce lower back problems, as well as fight general weakness, decreasing your risk of falls and fractures.

If you want to get into the swing of golf, remember these tips.

- Before you start playing, walk the course each day for a couple of weeks. It's a fine way to get used to the terrain.

- Find a driving range near you and visit it often. It's a good place to practice your golf swing.

- As part of the warm-up before any golf game, use your golf club as a stretching tool. Hold it horizontally in front of you, and, without arching your back, lift it skyward. Then bring it back down to shoulder height and gently rotate your upper body to the right and then the left.

- Start out with a shorter backswing, progressing to a full swing as you gain strength and range of motion in your back. However, you can significantly reduce your backswing without affecting your stroke.

- Concentrate on turning your hips as you swing. This will relieve your back and improve your form.

- Improve your golf grip with an old phone book. Open the phone book and moisten your fingertips. Using one hand, press down with your fingertips, and rip, crumple, and discard one page. Alternate hands. Continue doing this until your hands are tired.

  You should be able to do more pages with your dominant hand. This exercise will improve grip strength, endurance, and flexibility.

- Chasing balls into the woods can raise your risk of tick-borne infections. Consider taking an extra stroke instead. At the very least, wear long sleeves and insect repellent, and be sure to check yourself over for ticks after you retrieve the ball.

If golf isn't the only sport that interests you, that's good. Activities that improve your strength, aerobic fitness, and flexibility may help your golf game, too.

Stay young with healthy hobbies

"I've been playing tennis as long as I've been gardening," says 79-year-old Anne, a former landscape architect. "But I only took up croquet last year. And I love it because it's much more complicated than people think."

Croquet may be her newest passion, but gardening has been a lifelong love. Every April, Anne starts work on her flower garden. "The first couple of weeks are really hard," she admits. "But it's fun."

She has plenty of cleanup, trimming and planting to do, but Anne is savvy enough to pace herself. As she advises, "Don't try to tackle the whole thing the first day."

But to Anne, the results are worth the effort. "You have lovely flowers you can pick and enjoy in your house all year long. It's like good music."

Anne took up croquet because she thought joint pain might someday prevent her from playing tennis. "At least I can have something to do with other people. And it's a fun, *thinking* game," she says delightedly. "I never realized. It's not like the old croquet."

So far, Anne continues to play tennis several times a week. She wisely chooses doubles and plays on a soft court. "You meet an awful lot of people. If I didn't have tennis, I would have been an old couch potato and that's no good."

Occasionally, tennis can be a good way to vent frustrations, too. "When you're mad," Anne explains, "boy, you can slam the ball and get it out of your system."

Anne has a tip for folks who worry that they can't keep moving. "If they used to play tennis – they can do it again," she declares. "It's all in the mind. You've got to be an 'I can' person instead of an 'I can't' person."

Serve up fitness fun with tennis

You want fitness benefits? Try taking it to court – a tennis court, that is. Grab a tennis racket and see how many advantages you can rack up.

Tennis is a game you play on an indoor or outdoor court. Here's how it works. A net divides the court in half down the center. Opponents stand on opposite sides of the net and hit the ball back and forth. The object, of course, is to place the ball within certain boundaries but so your opponent cannot hit the ball back to you.

There's a good deal of running and swinging and hitting involved – at least in singles tennis. If you play doubles, you have two people on each side of the net and no one has to run quite as hard or fast to hit the ball.

Although you need to learn more about tennis before you can play, you can see how tennis could give you a workout.

According to the American Academy of Family Physicians, playing racket sports regularly may help slow or prevent the bone loss linked to osteoporosis.

Don Schroer is a former tennis coach and current Chairman of Health, Physical Education, and Dance at Emory University. He explains how tennis and fitness go together.

"Balance, flexibility, coordination, and agility are the basic components of the game," he explains. "Players maintain and develop these through play, drill work, and a balanced conditioning program." That means strength training, stretches, and aerobic exercise should improve your tennis game.

Tennis can work the muscles in your arms, legs, and midriff. Although it's also good for your heart and lungs, Schroer says that tennis may not be the perfect aerobic workout.

"Because of the stop and go nature of the sport and the numerous rest periods between points or games, I don't think tennis would rank as the number one aerobic activity," he says. But he adds that players need to be in good aerobic shape for matches that run long. "This is not only a game of skill, but also a game of physical endurance," he explains.

"Tennis as an exercise routine is also a great mental stress release," Schroer points out. He adds that many people play because they enjoy the social time with friends and colleagues.

At 41, Rachel has been playing tennis for over a decade – and she credits the sport with introducing her to some good friends. "I love the strategy, competition and friendships tennis brings to my life," she says. "I have a desk job and love the chance to get outside and do something physical and totally opposite of my work. Tennis gives me that opportunity."

If you'd like to try tennis, here are some tips to keep in mind.

- If you've never played tennis before, take lessons to learn the rules.

- Although you may spend some money on a tennis racket and balls, you don't have to pay much to play. In the city where Rachel lives, she can play on any one of 40 outdoor courts in parks or at the local university – all at little or no cost.

- Rachel says a tennis match can last from two to two and one-half hours. If that's too long to play the more strenuous one-on-one game of singles tennis, try doubles. You won't wear yourself out as quickly, but you can still have fun and get fit.

If tennis isn't quite right for you, consider other racket sports. The American Heart Association recommends both badminton and table tennis as excellent choices for older adults.

Calculate the ways to burn calories

Here's something to think about when choosing between fitness options. According to the Calorie Control Council, the following chart shows how many calories a 150-pound person would burn by doing a particular activity for just 30 minutes.

If you want to burn more calories, consider those activities higher up in the chart. Of course you should check with your doctor before trying any new exercise or sport. But, if your doctor approves, you may have extra fun while you watch pounds slip away.

Whether you want to burn calories or just have a great time getting fit, always remember that having fun helps fire up more enthusiasm for your fitness plan. On top of that, fun may help you stay committed to exercise even if your willpower gives out. So put the ideas in this chapter to work – and keep an eagle eye out for new things to try. You'll get more fun out of fitness and your body will thank you for it.

Fitness Activity	Calories Burned
Jogging	338
Swimming	302
Tennis (singles)	275
Weightlifting	234
Bicycling (no hills)	221
Racquetball	221
Aerobics	203
Badminton (singles)	198
Walking (briskly)	198
Scrubbing floors	189
Yoga	180
Tennis (doubles)	171
Ballroom dancing	153
Washing a car	153
Walking a dog	149
Water aerobics	144
Swing dancing	135
Table tennis	135
Tai chi	135
Golfing (no cart)	131
Grocery shopping	122
Strolling	104
Vacuuming	85

Go for the gold

Do you need a challenge to keep the fun in fitness? If you're over 50, you could go for gold at the National Senior Games.

Around 10,000 senior athletes plan to compete in 18 sports at the next Summer National Senior Games. In many events, there are several age groups, with a gold medal for the winner in each. So what kind of games do senior Olympians play?

■ Ball sports include basketball, bowling, golf, racquetball, softball, tennis, table tennis, and volleyball.

■ Other summer events are archery, badminton, cycling, horseshoes, race walking, road racing, shuffleboard, swimming, triathlon, and track and field sports.

For local, state, or national information, contact the National Senior Games Association. Visit their Web site <www.nsga.com> or write them at:

P.O. Box 82059
Baton Rouge, LA 70884-2059

The inside scoop on diet dangers

13

Weigh in on the side of good health

You may notice natural changes in your weight now that you have started exercising and following a nutritious eating plan. If you are still not at your ideal weight, however, there are some good reasons to take off a few more pounds.

Lighten up, for health's sake

You look good and feel energetic when you maintain a trim figure, but your health is an even more important reason to watch your weight.

Doctors used to think after age 55 people didn't gain and, in fact, gradually lost pounds. But that doesn't hold true. Obesity, or excess body fat, is growing faster among seniors than any other group.

Experts say extra weight hurts your health even more than smoking or heavy drinking. It increases your risk for diabetes, heart disease, stroke, high blood pressure, gallbladder disease, sleep apnea and other breathing problems, osteoarthritis, and some forms of cancer. But the good news is, you can do something about it.

If you are overweight, starting on a healthy weight-loss plan now may add years to your life. In fact, one study found that just trying to lose – even if you don't succeed – can help you live longer. That may be because, in an effort to reduce your weight, you are likely to eat more nutritious foods and practice a healthier lifestyle in other ways, too.

4 clues it's time to take off pounds

You may wonder if the weight you've added over the years is enough to affect your health. Here are some ways to find out.

Compare apples and pears. Look in the mirror and note where your extra weight is located. Fat stored around your waistline is much more dangerous to your health than fat stored on your hips and thighs.

In fact, fat around your waist, giving you an apple shape, puts you at higher risk for heart disease than if a few extra pounds have settled in the lower part of your body, giving you a pear-shaped appearance.

Measure your middle. Just how much girth is a problem? Consider your health at risk if you are a woman with a waist measurement of more than 35 inches. If you are a man, 40 inches or more means it's time to reduce.

Even with a smaller measurement, you may still be at risk for health problems if your waistline has increased 2 inches or more since you've reached maturity.

Check the charts. Use the body mass index (BMI) chart to determine the ratio of your weight to your height. This will help you decide if your weight is in a healthy range. A BMI between 19 and 25 is considered healthy. A BMI above 25 generally means you are overweight, and over 30 indicates you are obese, a more serious health concern.

This index is based on the assumption that having extra weight means you have more body fat. If, however, you are muscular you may fall into an overweight category but still be healthy.

As you get older, waist measurement may be a more accurate indicator of obesity than BMI. Many seniors lose muscle mass as they gain fat. That means it's possible to fall within the healthy weight category when, in fact, you're carrying too much unhealthy fat.

Get expert advice. Not all seniors should go on a diet. Talk to your doctor, especially if you are over 65 or plan to lose more than 20 pounds. Be sure to discuss the cause of your weight gain, and find out how other health conditions – like diabetes and high blood pressure – come into play.

Body mass index (BMI) chart

Weight Height	100	110	120	130	140	150	160	170	180	190	200
5'0"	20	21	23	25	27	29	31	33	35	37	39
5'1"	19	21	23	25	26	28	30	32	34	36	38
5'2"	18	20	22	24	26	27	29	31	33	35	37
5'3"	18	19	21	23	25	27	28	30	32	34	35
5'4"	17	19	21	22	24	26	27	29	31	33	34
5'5"	17	18	20	22	23	25	27	28	30	32	33
5'6"	16	18	19	21	23	24	26	27	29	31	32
5'7"	16	17	19	20	22	23	25	27	28	30	31
5'8"	15	17	18	20	21	23	24	26	27	29	30
5'9"	15	16	18	19	21	22	24	25	27	28	30
5'10"	14	16	17	19	20	22	23	24	26	27	29
5'11"	14	15	17	18	20	21	22	24	25	26	28
6'0"	14	15	16	18	19	20	22	23	24	26	27
6'1"	13	15	16	17	18	20	21	22	24	25	26
6'2"	13	14	15	17	18	19	21	22	23	24	26
6'3"	12	14	15	16	17	19	20	21	22	24	25

Don't fall for dangerous diet frauds

You want to lose some weight, and you want to lose it now. So those advertisements for diets, pills, body wraps, patches, and creams really catch your attention. It's hard to resist their promises – no matter how unbelievable they may sound.

Fantastic guarantees, however, should be your first clue that the claims may not be trustworthy. If it's too easy – like swallowing a "calorie blocker" or a "fat magnet" pill before you eat – it is too good to be true.

And don't be fooled by a name that seems reliable – like the Mayo Clinic Diet, for example. The truth is, the Mayo Clinic has never given its backing to a grapefruit diet, an egg diet, or any of the many other quick weight-loss plans that use their name.

Quick-fix diets waste your money and delay getting started on a nutritious eating plan. If you do lose weight, you are likely to gain it back quickly. Worse still, are diet pills, which can be a deadly mistake. Unfortunately, almost everybody is tempted to take them when they want to get rid of weight fast.

Remember that fen-phen was taken off the market because it caused heart damage. And phenylpropanolamine (PPA) is an ingredient in some diet pills which makes blood pressure shoot dangerously high. Now the FDA proposes a mandatory warning label on all products containing ephedra, or ma huang. There's evidence it causes heart attacks, strokes, and seizures. In fact, some manufacturers are voluntarily withdrawing diet supplements containing ephedra.

It seems as fast as one dangerous diet pill is taken off the market, an untested substitute is there to take its place. Bitter orange, or *Citrus aurantium*, is a current favorite. It's harmless in small amounts as a flavoring for food, but contains a compound, synephrine, that works in much the same way as ephedra.

Experts believe the amounts of bitter orange used in over-the-counter supplements can raise your blood pressure and cause heart problems, especially if used in combination with other stimulants, like caffeine. And it can interact with certain prescription medications.

But here's the good news. A healthy eating and lifestyle program like the one outlined in this book, will help you lose weight safely and keep it off for the rest of your life.

Beware the perils of popular diets

That slender actress sounds so convincing when she sings the praises of the latest Hollywood diet. But a testimonial from a movie star is not the same thing as solid advice from a health professional.

Experts agree you can lose weight on many of the fad diets. That's because you'll eat fewer calories – although that fact may be hidden in the advertising hype. Unfortunately on most of these diets, you will cut out important nutrients as you cut calories.

Success story: from heavyweight to fitness pro

Pat Burton has tried a lot of diets.

"I remember eating nothing but 6 cups of cooked rice with fake butter and a pint of salsa poured over the top," he says. "I did the same thing with corn. And I wondered why I wasn't losing any weight!"

Pat was 40 years old and "a biscuit away from 300 pounds," he recalls, when he decided it was time to change his eating patterns. A year later, with the help of a nutritionist plus his own research, he's 100 pounds lighter with 20 percent less body fat.

"I didn't recreate the wheel or do anything earth-shattering," he says modestly. "I just got serious about my health and started by making little changes that snowballed into major lifestyle changes."

Pat's old pattern was to skip breakfast and lunch, eat lots of snacks during the day, and finish with a big dinner at night. White rice, pasta, and potatoes were a large part of his diet.

Now his meals are low in fat, but higher in protein and fruits and vegetables. He chooses whole-grain bread and brown rice over highly processed grains. He has six or seven small meals a day, and stops eating at least three hours before bedtime.

Keeping a diary was an important part of Pat's success. "It initially was my conscience," he says. "Knowing if I ate something I would have to record it and look at it later kept me honest."

Pat, now a cycling enthusiast and fitness instructor, believes just eating right wasn't enough. "Exercise had to be there," he says, "for it all to come together."

Diet losses don't always last

The problem with popular diets is they are designed for one purpose – to help you lose weight. But if they don't teach you to change your eating patterns for the rest of your life, the weight will return. This yo-yo dieting – losing, gaining back, losing again, gaining back again – can lead to health problems.

According to nutritionists, if you are an average-size person and you consistently eat about 1,400 to 1,500 calories a day, no matter how much physical activity you get, you will probably lose weight. You may need to adjust that number up or down a little if you are taller and more muscular or smaller than most.

Dietitian Dawn Jackson, a spokesperson for the American Dietetic Association (ADA) says, "In general, we know a 1,500-calorie diet is good for weight loss and you don't have to go much lower."

Counting calories isn't enough

So why not just pick a diet that meets this calorie requirement and follow it? Experts like Jackson believe there's more to it than that.

"These diets do work in the short run," she says, "but they won't work for the long haul. We aren't interested in people just losing weight. We want to help people lose weight and keep it off."

So you won't sacrifice your health, you must pay attention to nutrition. According to the National Academy of Sciences, a healthy eating plan has the following breakdown of total calories:

■ 45 - 65 percent should come from carbohydrates

■ 10 - 35 percent should come from protein

■ 20 - 35 percent should come from fats

A healthy weight-loss plan should stay within these ranges, but shouldn't rule out any single food. Most fad diets are based on good foods and bad foods. Jackson says this sabotages your success. Not only are they nutritionally unbalanced, they are also hard to stick to if they don't allow some of your favorite foods.

How the 'in' diets do harm

Everybody seems to have a favorite diet-of-the-month. And each one has its pros and cons. But here's the real scoop on some of the most popular plans.

High-protein diets. The Atkins Diet is the best-known protein-packed weight-loss plan – also called low-carbohydrate or high-fat diets. Others you may hear about are The Carbohydrate Addict's Diet, a Sugar Busters diet, and The Protein Power Lifeplan.

Initially these may sound like a good way to lose. You can load up on all the meat, cheese, eggs, and other high-fat foods you want, so you aren't likely to go hungry.

Unfortunately, you're allowed few fruits, vegetables, or whole grains. And – according to the American Heart Association and others – you may be putting your health in danger. Here are a few of the reasons.

- Too much protein can cause your body to get rid of calcium, leaving your bones weak and brittle. It also puts a strain on your kidneys, making a high-protein diet especially dangerous for diabetics. It can also lead to gout.

- A lot of saturated fat, the kind that causes cholesterol buildup in your arteries, comes with many high-protein foods. So while you may lose weight, your risk for heart disease and stroke could increase.

  Recent research hasn't found this to be as big a problem as feared, but none of the studies focused on people older than 53, nor did they look at what happens if you stay on the diet long-term. Therefore, many health experts still aren't convinced a high protein diet is safe.

- When you limit fruits, vegetables, and whole grains, you eliminate natural ways to lower your blood pressure and fight cancer. You also open the door to vitamin and mineral deficiencies.

- A low-carbohydrate diet removes your main source of energy. The result – you are fatigued after exercising, and your body must burn muscle tissue for energy.

Another popular diet, The Zone, touts a 40-30-30 ratio of carbohydrates, protein, and fats, about double the protein other experts recommend.

In addition, many of The Zone's biochemical claims have never been proven – like the theory eating fat will not cause your body to store more fat.

Many people find it hard to stay with diets like these which limit the kinds of foods you can eat. They get boring pretty quickly. And they definitely don't teach you long-term healthy eating habits.

Very-low-fat diets. At the opposite extreme from the high-protein diets are the very-low-fat diets. These have been popular for years. But while the amount of fat people eat has dropped in the last two decades, obesity in the U.S. has doubled.

According to Jackson, low-fat diets continue to be the favorite with seniors. "They tend to be fearful of beef and eggs," she says, "even good fats like olive oil and nuts."

But cutting out too much fat isn't in your best interest. Here's why.

■ Your body needs some fat to produce hormones and bile and to carry certain fat-soluble vitamins through your bloodstream.

And when you cut out fat you usually reduce protein as well since they are often found together in meats, cheese, and other foods. Your body needs some protein to keep your muscles from breaking down and to repair skin, tendons, ligaments, hair and other tissues.

■ Low-fat doesn't necessarily mean low-calorie. A lot of people on low-fat diets discover they aren't losing weight.

The truth is, fat-free cookies, cakes, and other treats may sabotage your best weight-loss efforts. These foods are often loaded with sugar, flour, and starch thickeners to make them taste better. In fact, they may have more calories than the full-fat versions.

It's not just the sweets you need to watch out for. If you fill up on white bread and bagels, polished rice, and fat-free chips, the calories can still creep up before you know it. There's some evidence that eating these quick-release refined carbs makes you hungrier.

These are good reasons to stick to fruits, vegetables and whole grains – carbs that are dense in nutrients and fiber, and digest more slowly.

■ Even if you eat plenty of lean protein and go for the healthy carbs, Jackson believes something is still missing.

"You can definitely get enough fruits, vegetables, and whole grains from a very-low-fat diet, and that's healthy," she says. "But a lot of times it's satisfaction that is missing – and some good fats, like from nuts and fish."

Dean Ornish's low-fat diet was designed to help people reverse heart disease. That would seem to make it a good diet for everyone, right?

"For the general population – even for people interested in reversing heart disease – it can be very hard to follow for the long term," says Jackson. This seems to be true, she believes, at either extreme end of the spectrum.

Extreme calorie restriction. You may lose weight fastest on very-low-calorie diets. "But," Jackson says, "it is very difficult to have human beings get all their nutrition if they are eating less than 1,200 calories a day."

And while reducing calories is essential in your battle to slim down, hunger is the factor most likely to defeat you. At a slower pace, with one pound per week as your weight-loss goal, you can have enough healthy food to satisfy your hunger.

Ultra-low-calorie diets – 800 calories a day or less – should be considered only in very special circumstances and then solely with your doctor's supervision.

Prepackaged programs have pros and cons

It's possible to get balanced nutrition and lose weight on Weight Watchers and Jenny Craig, two of the most popular plans organized around prepackaged meals.

What Jackson recommends about these depends on the personality, lifestyle, and financial circumstances of the individual she's counseling.

"Jenny Craig," she says, "may be good for a person who has money and wants the convenience of proportioned, prepackaged food." Jackson emphasizes, however, that it won't teach a person about foods and nutrition over the long-term.

And what about Weight Watchers? "It's good for someone who loves to keep logs and likes the accountability of weekly meetings," says Jackson.

Calories aren't always the culprit

If you stick to a moderate diet, but the pounds still pile on, there could be another — although rare — explanation for your weight gain. Ask your doctor if one of these could be the cause.

- **Hypothyroidism.** If your thyroid produces too little thyroid hormone, your metabolism slows down and you gain weight. If this is your problem, you may often feel cold and fatigued. You need to have a blood test to check it out.

- **Genetics.** You may have inherited a condition that contributes to weight gain — like not enough of a particular hormone that signals when you are full.

- **Medications.** Estrogen, some antidepressants, and several other drugs can cause weight gain. Don't stop taking your meds, just talk to your doctor or pharmacist about an alternative prescription.

20-20-20:
your winning
weight-loss plan

14

20 steps to weight loss

Are you ready to lose 20 pounds in 20 weeks and feel as energetic as you did 20 years ago? You can't go wrong with this 20-20-20 weight-loss plan – perhaps the last diet you'll ever need.

The 20 easy-to-follow steps are based on solid scientific research and sound advice from doctors and nutrition experts.

■ Step 1: Begin with a commitment to good health

The earlier chapter – *Nutrition know-how* – may have inspired you to follow its suggested eating plan. If so, you've probably already noticed a difference in how you feel and you may have lost some weight, as well. If you haven't taken its 8-week nutrition plan to heart, go back and read that chapter again. Make those changes a part of your routine for at least a month. This will lay a strong foundation for the 20-20-20 weight-loss plan.

■ Step 2: Prepare yourself mentally

Losing weight permanently and safely is a life-changing concept. Think about the good reasons for wanting to lose weight – better health, more energy, improved appearance. Be sure it's your idea, not someone else's.

■ Step 3: Build a support network

Let family and friends know your intention. Spend time with those who encourage you, and avoid those who would throw cold water on your plan.

■ Step 4: Set realistic goals

For most, a goal of one pound per week – 20 pounds in 20 weeks – is ideal. This may seem like a modest goal, but it's best over the long term. Losing weight slowly but steadily means the weight is more likely to stay off. And certain health problems, like gallstones, can develop if you lose weight too fast. Two pounds per week is the absolute most you should consider losing unless, for health reasons, your doctor supervises you on a quicker plan.

■ Step 5: Keep a food diary

Begin with awareness of what you really are eating – not what you think you are eating – by writing it all down.

"Although people will always fight it, keeping a food diary improves self-awareness," says Dawn Jackson, Chicago dietitian and spokesperson for the American Dietetic Association. "We know from the National Weight Registry of thousands of people who have lost weight and kept it off, successful dieters monitor their food intake along with their weight."

You'll find a blank meal diary on the next page. Use it to log the foods you eat and the number of calories in each. There's a helpful food and calories list later in this chapter, but you can use any calorie counter. Write down every calorie – don't be tempted to fudge. You're the only one who needs to see this, and if it isn't accurate it won't be helpful.

■ Step 6: Decide your daily calorie limit

After recording your calories for one week, add together your seven daily totals and divide that number by 7. This will give you the average calories you are eating each day.

No matter what the creators of fad diets say, the most important thing weight-loss champs know – and you should, too – is that to lose weight you must burn more calories than you take in. And to lose one pound per week, you need to cut out 500 calories each day.

So, subtract 500 calories from your daily average, and you'll see how many calories you can eat a day and still meet your weight-loss goal.

Meal Diary (calculate how many calories you normally eat each day, then find your daily average)

	Monday	Tuesday	Wednesday	Thursday	Friday	Saturday	Sunday
	Breakfast	Breakfast	Breakfast	Breakfast	Breakfast	Breakfast	Breakfast
	Calories:	Calories:	Calories:	Calories:	Calories:	Calories:	Calories:
	Lunch	Lunch	Lunch	Lunch	Lunch	Lunch	Lunch
	Calories:	Calories:	Calories:	Calories:	Calories:	Calories:	Calories:
	Dinner	Dinner	Dinner	Dinner	Dinner	Dinner	Dinner
	Calories:	Calories:	Calories:	Calories:	Calories:	Calories:	Calories:
	Snacks	Snacks	Snacks	Snacks	Snacks	Snacks	Snacks
	Calories:	Calories:	Calories:	Calories:	Calories:	Calories:	Calories:
	Total	Total	Total	Total	Total	Total	Total

Add up your daily totals to get your weekly total calories:

Average daily calorie intake: _____ ÷ by 7

■ Step 7: Make a meal plan

Base your daily menus on the number of calories you just calculated. Choose nutrient-dense foods, as opposed to those with empty calories, and remember to get the recommended number of servings from each food group.

As you plan your own meals, be aware of calorie density, too. Carbohydrates and proteins have about four calories per gram, while fat has nine calories – more than twice as many – per gram. So you can fill up on bulky grains and vegetables, for example, and get far fewer calories than from the same amount of fatty meats and desserts.

Spread your calories throughout the day. Munching more often on smaller meals will help you lose weight without feeling hungry. Use the sample eating plans you'll find later in this chapter to get started. They provide three primary meals and two "mini meals," or snacks, for three different calorie levels.

■ Step 8: Measure your portions

The actual amounts of food you eat are often different from – and larger than – standard serving sizes. For a while use measuring cups and spoons to check the size of your portions, at least until you learn to "eyeball" what a serving really is.

This will help you more accurately calculate the calories you are actually eating. It will also help show if you are getting all the recommended servings of the different food groups. Read labels on prepared foods for serving sizes.

To get the best balance of nutrients while staying in your calorie range, Jackson suggests you re-proportion the food on a typical plate. Think of a three-portion picnic plate, and place a starch – like brown rice – and a protein – maybe fish or chicken – in the smaller sections. Fill the larger space with vegetables, which, as a rule, are high in nutrients and low in calories.

■ Step 9: Don't skip meals

If you want to lose weight fast, your first thought may be to cut out a few meals. But hunger pangs can send you searching desperately for something – anything – to eat. Keeping to a regular schedule is the best way to assure you won't get or stay hungry.

Above all, don't forget to eat breakfast. Nutritionists say it can play a major role in the long-term success of your weight-loss plan.

■ Step 10: Determine your eating weaknesses

Everybody has them – those foods you just can't resist. The best way to manage those cravings is to allow small indulgences from time to time.

Of course, it's best if your favorite treat also has some health benefit. Although an ounce of dark chocolate, for example, has about 150 calories, it may be good for your heart. If cookies are your weakness, consider those that are fruit-filled, like Fig Newtons. They provide lots of fiber and antioxidant nutrients.

If torn between a sweet beverage and a dessert, go for the solid. In one study, people who ate a sweet snack were less hungry and ate less at the next meal, than those who drank a sugary drink with the same number of calories.

■ Step 11: Recognize emotional eating triggers

Some people clean house when they are angry. Others can't seem to stop eating when they are bored, sad, or lonely. To guard against binge eating at times of emotional stress, try these four steps.

Figure out why the craving hits. Record in your food diary not only what you eat and how much, but also when, where, and what you are feeling. Knowing what events trigger eating sprees helps you prevent them.

Think of things you could do instead of eating. Go for a walk or a bike ride, put on some music and dance out your frustrations, or call up a friend who will be a supportive listener.

Give in occasionally. If you haven't allowed yourself a favorite comfort food lately – or at least a satisfying substitute – it may be harder to resist over-indulging when stress hits. Letting yourself savor a small dish of your favorite ice cream may be just what the doctor ordered for your mental and emotional health.

Replace junk food with healthy choices. If you only have wholesome, low-calorie treats available, when the desire to binge hits you won't be able to do much damage. Keep a piece of fruit or a bag of baby carrots and other vegetable munchies handy, wherever you are.

▪ Step 12: Take a supplement

Although foods are your best source of nutrients, when you lower your calories, it's a good idea to back up even the most nutritious diet with a daily multiple vitamin and mineral pill.

▪ Step 13: Exercise to burn calories

You will drop some pounds by dropping calories, but if you want to keep the weight off, you've got to exercise. You'll also reduce stress, which can contribute to weight gain. These are two rules you must follow.

Many experts believe walking is your best exercise choice. According to some studies, it may actually be more effective for trimming down than running or other popular physical activities. Since you are less prone to injury when walking, you are less likely to become an exercise dropout.

▪ Step 14: Rest well

At the end of a difficult day, you may wonder if you'll be able to hold to your new calorie goal. But after a good night's sleep your confidence should bounce back. One study suggests that willpower returns after rest, or a positive emotional experience.

▪ Step 15: Dine out with care

Don't avoid restaurants because you're trying to lose weight – just have a plan, or the menu will sabotage your best intentions. These tips should help you enjoy the experience and stick to your calorie count.

Opt for lunch. The portions are generally smaller than at dinner.

Go light. Choose a restaurant with "light" dishes on the menu. Or call ahead to see if they will make adjustments, like grilling an item that's usually fried or substituting steamed vegetables for French fries.

Divide and conquer. Ask for a take-out container at the beginning rather than the end of a meal. Fill it with half your food – two-thirds if they serve extra-large portions – before you begin to eat. You can divide it again when you get home then freeze or refrigerate it for later meals.

Skip the entrées. Instead make your meal from a salad, broth-based soup, and a low-calorie appetizer – like shrimp cocktail.

Ban the buffet. If you can't avoid an all-you-can-eat food bar, limit yourself to two trips. Load up a dinner plate with fruits, salads, and other low-calorie vegetable dishes. If you eat it all and still want more, use a small salad plate for the second visit.

Allow sensible treats. When a pizza craving hits, order a veggie special on thin crust with double tomato sauce and a light sprinkling of cheese.

■ Step 16: Weigh in weekly

Slow but steady weight loss can seem discouraging on a daily basis. Since your weight can change slightly as your body holds and loses water during the day, a weekly reading will be more accurate.

■ Step 17: Reward yourself

You'll keep your enthusiasm high if you celebrate small successes. Treat yourself to a massage, go to a movie, or spend time with friends in an activity, like hiking, that doesn't include food. And you can always throw out your old clothes and reward yourself with new smaller ones!

■ Step 18: Avoid setbacks

It's less likely you'll stumble on the path to a trimmer, healthier you if you have a clear plan. This must include an emergency strategy.

Holiday season, for example, is usually a "code red" – when your careful eating routine is bushwhacked. Think ahead and go to a maintenance level plan (see next step) for those times when losing weight will temporarily be more difficult.

Don't get discouraged if you do have a setback. Acknowledge it happened, put it behind you, and recommit to your plan. "Aim for progress and not perfection," says Jackson.

■ Step 19: Establish a maintenance plan

When you reach your weight-loss goal, slowly increase your calories. Over a month, allow about 100 more daily calories during the first two weeks and another 100 the next two weeks.

You'll probably need to add back in fewer total calories than the 500 you originally cut. That's because you are a smaller person now and your body needs fewer calories to function. So check your weight weekly as you add calories back. Add more if you continue to lose weight – and don't want to – but cut back a little if you start gaining.

■ **Step 20: Rest at your new level**

Maintain your new weight for a few months, enjoying your success, before you decide if you need to lose any more. If you find you are ready to drop a few more pounds, go back to the fourth step and set a new goal.

Drink from the fountain of youth

When you've successfully reached your weight-loss goal with the 20-20-20 plan, your next objective might be to live to be 100. Dr. Roy Walford, author of *The Anti-Aging Plan* and *Beyond the 120-Year Diet,* thinks that's a reasonable notion.

Walford believes to extend your potential life span — the number of years you are likely to live — you must deeply and permanently reduce your calories. And to stay healthy and mentally sharp throughout your longer life, all those calories should be jam-packed with nutrition.

Follow his anti-aging diet, Walford says, and you can substantially reduce your risk of most diseases that usually plague your middle and late years.

His plan calls for gradual weight loss over six months to about a year. Then if you eat correctly, you can maintain your new "weight point" with your body operating at top efficiency and health.

Walford's books provide menus, recipes, and strict advice about working with your doctor.

---

20 tips for a successful shape-up

Sometimes it's the little things that trip you up on you path to your healthiest, most ideal weight. Avoid those pitfalls by backing up your 20-20-20 plan with these helpful tips.

- **Make a smooth start.** Stress can wreck your best intentions. So if you are starting a new job, getting a divorce, or there has been a recent death in your family, you might need to delay your plan. Give yourself more time to simply follow good eating habits without trying to lose. Then, when the stress has eased, you'll be ready to start cutting back on calories.

- **Choose a traditional dining spot.** Make it a habit to sit down and eat at a table – not in the car, not at your desk at work, and not "on the run."

- **Dine amid soft or neutral colors.** Bright colors stimulate the appetite, so choose calmer tones in tablecloths, napkins, and even dining room walls. Turning up the lights, on the other hand, may help you avoid overeating. One researcher found people ate more in a darkened room.

- **Pick a perfect plate.** Use a small dinner plate – the same size every meal. Helpings look larger on the smaller space, so you are less likely to overload or feel deprived. In addition, you'll need less measuring as you learn what a single serving of various foods looks like on your dish.

- **Take your time.** Chew slowly and put down your fork between bites. Your brain needs 20 minutes to get the message your hunger is satisfied.

- **Play mellow music.** Listening to soft classical music, according to one study, helps you eat less – and more slowly. But snappier rock and roll may cause you to eat more and faster.

- **Stop eating when you're satisfied.** When you reach that "had enough" feeling, put down your fork, get up from the table, put away leftovers, and get busy with something other than eating.

- **Stock up on healthy foods.** Go through your pantry and refrigerator and remove any junk food you find. Restock your shelves with nutritious, low-calorie substitutes.

- **Calm down before you chow down.** Don't turn to food to relieve tensions. If you are having a stressful day, go for a walk, meditate, or listen to soothing music to calm yourself before eating. You'll be less likely to overindulge.

■ **Visualize success.** Relax and use imagery each day to get a feel for victory. See yourself, having already reached your goal, slipping into a smaller-sized outfit. Or imagine feeling proud as you step on your bathroom scale and see the numbers. Pretending it's already true enlists the support of your subconscious mind to make it really happen.

■ **Take up a new – or rediscover an old – hobby.** Choose a pastime like knitting or cross-stitching. Hook a rug, put a puzzle together, or place family photos in an album. Not only will you keep your hands too busy to reach for a snack, you'll also get the satisfaction of completing a task.

■ **Measure your treats.** Don't nibble from a bag or box, especially while watching television or using the computer. When you are distracted you are likely to eat more than you planned. Instead, measure a small amount – like a handful of pretzels or a couple of cookies – and put the rest away. Give your full attention to slowly eating your snack before you return to your activity.

■ **Drink up and freeze out fat.** Some diet pros say drinking a big glass of ice water before meals will dull your appetite. Liquids of any temperature make you feel fuller. Plus, sometimes people eat when they are really just thirsty. So pour a glass of water instead of reaching for something to nibble. If plain water seems boring, add a twist of lemon or drink flavored bottled water or unsweetened herbal iced tea.

■ **Juice your way to a slim, trim figure.** Delicious, vitamin-filled orange juice – or another fructose-rich juice – may be the perfect appetizer for anyone trying to lose weight. In a Yale study, those who drank a 200-calorie glass of juice half an hour or so before eating cut calories at mealtime – from 300 to more than 400 on average. Stir in a little pectin, which is used to thicken jams and jellies, and you may reduce your appetite even more.

■ **Be positive about "negative" calories.** Celery, cucumbers, and iceberg lettuce have very few calories. In fact, some people call them "negative-calorie" foods because, they say, in preparing, chewing, and digesting them, you burn more calories than they contain.

Whether this is true or not, snack away on them until you are as thin as you want to be.

■ **Eat light at night for a flat tummy.** You may have heard that eating a big meal late at night isn't a good idea – whether you want to lose weight or just sleep well. But did you know this habit could give you a potbelly? That's because a heavy meal puts pressure on your stomach muscles and pushes them out. It does this more easily when these muscles are relaxed, as they are when you lie down to sleep. A "bay window" is the result if this happens regularly.

Worrying about your weight can also contribute to a bulging midsection. Studies show stress seems to cause fat to settle around the waist – a dangerous place to carry it, as you know. Exercise, however, is helpful for both reducing stress and keeping pounds off. Try to hold you stomach muscles in when you walk, run, or do other exercises that bounce your belly. The flopping motion can weaken those abdominal muscles.

■ **Shop with a list.** Plan your meals carefully before you make your shopping list. Then stick to it while you are in the store. Don't linger in the aisles where you might be tempted to buy extras. Watch out, especially, for yummy-sounding names. Grandma's Oven-Fresh Old-Fashioned Oatmeal Cookies, for example, are probably plain oatmeal cookies, mass-produced in a commercial bakery. Remind yourself they are nothing special and go back to your list.

■ **Read the labels.** You'll learn a lot by reading the information on packages in the store. Better yet, many companies provide nutrition data – including calories – online. So surf for the facts before you make your shopping list.

■ **Don't shop when you are hungry or rushed.** Have a healthy, filling snack before you go out the door. The free food samples won't look so appetizing, and you'll be less tempted to buy unplanned extras from tantalizing displays.

If you make it a leisurely shopping trip, you'll have time to compare brands for the lowest calories per serving. And you can wait for the butcher to trim excess fat from the meats you buy.

■ **Feast on foods that force weight loss.** High fiber fruits, vegetables, and grains are your most nutritious weight-loss foods. They eliminate snacking by filling your tummy with the fewest calories at mealtime. The fiber makes you feel so full, in fact, it's as if someone turned off your body's internal hunger switch. Moreover, most fiber actually passes through your system undigested, so you don't absorb all the calories. And it does all this while lowering your cholesterol and blood pressure.

8 secret fiber-rich foods

Flaxseed. This tiny, nutritious seed may be the #1 weight-loss food. What's more, it protects your heart, eases arthritis, battles diabetes, and boosts your immune system. Grind flaxseed for best absorption, and sprinkle it on cereals or salads, bake it in breads, and stir it into sauces and stews.

Potatoes. Boil or bake them in their skins. Leave off the butter, and top them, instead, with salsa or fat-free sour cream and chives. One medium potato has about 160 calories and 4 grams of fiber.

Beans. Bake some great northerns or cook a pot of lentils. It takes a long time to absorb these high-fiber foods, so you'll feel full longer.

Whole-grain bread. Whole-wheat, for example, is much tastier, and more nutritious and filling than white bread.

Popcorn. Don't reach for a candy bar when this healthy low-calorie snack fills you up and keeps you satisfied longer.

Apples. Munch on an unpeeled MacIntosh — or another favorite — for a tasty alternative to low-fiber snacks.

Oranges. They fill you up more than bananas, and the whole fruit provides more fiber than orange juice.

Brown rice. This unprocessed grain gives you far more fiber than you'll find in white rice or pasta.These high-fiber foods also help prevent constipation. It's important, however, to drink lots of water with them. Otherwise, they might have the opposite effect.

Sample meals that slim and trim

You simply can't fail to lose weight if you carefully plan your meals around your target calorie level. To get started, look over the sample meal plans on the following pages. You'll find one for three different levels – 1,500 calories, 1,700 calories, and 1,900 calories. If your target doesn't match one of these numbers, just add or subtract food items or amounts.

Each plan includes three meals and two nutritious snacks. When an item is shown in italics and with an asterisk (*), that means you'll find the directions for making that dish in the recipe section.

If you don't care for an item on the sample plan, you can quickly use the food lists that follow the recipes to find a replacement with equal calories.

Just remember all you learned in the *Nutrition know-how* chapter about number of servings within food groups. The sample meal plans provide at least the minimum number of grains, fruits and vegetables, etc.

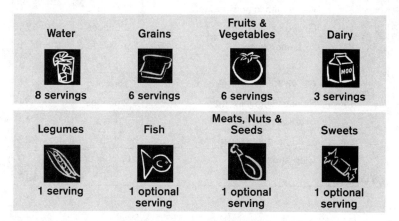

Water	Grains	Fruits & Vegetables	Dairy
8 servings	6 servings	6 servings	3 servings

Legumes	Fish	Meats, Nuts & Seeds	Sweets
1 serving	1 optional serving	1 optional serving	1 optional serving

You'll also find a blank form that you can photocopy for creating your own meal plans. Cross off servings at the bottom of it to help make sure you get the recommended number from each food group.

20-20-20 sample meal plan
1,500 calories per day

Meal	Food	Amount	Calories
Breakfast	Oatmeal with:	1 cup	122
	Raisins	1/4 cup	108
	Skim milk	1 cup	102
	Coffee	1 cup	5
Snack	Cantaloupe Crush*	1 serving	65
Lunch	Barley Lentil Soup*	1 serving	185
	Whole-wheat pita with:	1 small	74
	Avocado	1/2 medium	162
	Tomato	1 small	19
	Light Ranch dressing	1 tbl	38
	Frozen chocolate yogurt	1/2 cup	115
	Unsweetened brewed iced tea	12 ounces	3
Snack	Air-popped popcorn	1 cup	31
	Apple	1 medium	81
	Water with lemon wedge	8 ounces	1
Dinner	Grilled salmon with:	3 ounces	175
	Lemon juice	1 wedge	1
	Dill	1 tsp	3
	Get-To-Know-Your-Greens Salad*	1 serving	71
	Spinach linguini with:	2 ounces	74
	Olive oil	1 tsp	40
	Grated parmesan cheese	1 tbl	23
	Club soda	12 ounces	0
TOTAL			1,498

20-20-20 sample meal plan
1,700 calories per day

Meal	Food	Amount	Calories
Breakfast	Whole-wheat toast with:	2 slices	139
	Butter	2 pats	72
	Cinnamon	1 tsp	6
	Orange	1 large	86
	Coffee	1 cup	5
	Milk	1 cup	102
Snack	Multigrain brown rice cakes with:	2 cakes	70
	Apple butter	2 tbl	59
	Cantaloupe wedge	1/8 large	36
	Water with lemon wedge	8 ounces	1
Lunch	Romaine lettuce with:	2 cups	16
	Chopped green pepper	1/2 cup	20
	Chopped Italian tomato	1 medium	13
	Sliced ripe olives	10 large	51
	Flaxseed	1 tbl	59
	Fat-free Italian salad dressing	2 tbl	20
	Baked sweet potato with:	1 medium	117
	Butter	1 pat	36
	Brewed unsweetened iced tea	12 ounces	3
Snack	Plain whole milk yogurt with:	8 ounces	150
	Fresh blueberries	1/2 cup	14
	General Mills Fiber One cereal	1/2 cup	62
	Water with lemon wedge	8 ounces	1
Dinner	Grilled orange roughy with:	3 ounces	76
	Olive oil	1 tbl	119
	Caribbean Salsa*	1 serving	33
	Bountiful Black Bean Bulgur*	1 serving	147
	Vanilla soft-serve yogurt with:	1/2 cup	114
	Mini baking M&M's	1 tbl	73
	Club soda	12 ounces	0
TOTAL			1,700

20-20-20 sample meal plan
1,900 calories per day

Meal	Food	Amount	Calories
Breakfast	Bran flakes with:	1 cup	159
	Raisins	1/4 cup	109
	Flaxseed	1 tbl	59
	Skim milk	1 cup	100
	Coffee	1 cup	5
Snack	*Berry Power Drink**	1-1/2 cups	274
Lunch	Vegetable macaroni with:	1/2 cup	86
	Raw broccoli flowerets	1/4 cup	5
	Raw cauliflower flowerets	1/4 cup	6
	Chopped green pepper	1/4 cup	10
	Chopped tomato	1/4 cup	9
	Grated parmesan cheese	1 tbl	23
	Flaxseed	2 tbl	118
	Canned, drained kidney beans	1/2 cup	104
	Fat-free Italian salad dressing	2 tbl	20
	Low-salt wheat crackers	10 crackers	142
	Water with lemon wedge	8 ounces	1
Snack	Low-fat chocolate chip cookies	2 cookies	91
Dinner	*Ginger Sesame Alaska Salmon**	1 serving	252
	Brown rice	1/2 cup	109
	Angel food cake with:	1 serving	73
	Sliced fresh peaches	1 medium	42
	Low-fat vanilla yogurt	1/2 cup	105
	Water with lemon wedge	8 ounces	1
TOTAL			**1,903**

20-20-20 meal plan - _____ calories per day

Meal	Food	Amount	Calories
Breakfast			
Snack			
Lunch			
Snack			
Dinner			
TOTAL			

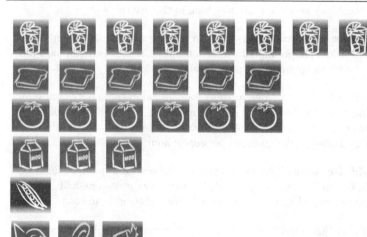

Optional

Recipes:
wholesome main meals

The recipes that follow make all the number-crunching easy. Each provides basic nutrition information to help you choose dishes that best fit your weight-loss plan and still please your taste buds.

You don't have to skip a savory-sounding recipe to meet special diet needs, either. If you're watching fat, cholesterol, sodium, or sugar, following these simple suggestions can make almost any meal fit your menu.

Reduce the fat. In general, muffins and quick breads can get by with one to two tablespoons of fat per cup of flour, while cakes take about two tablespoons per cup of flour. Here's another tip – soft drop cookies tend to have less fat than rolled cookies.

Cut the cholesterol. Replace whole eggs with egg whites when possible – two egg whites equal one egg – and follow the tips above for limiting fat. Many fatty foods are also high in cholesterol.

Skip the sodium. Buy low-sodium versions of ingredients, and cut the salt in baked recipes in half. Keep in mind yeast breads require around one-fourth teaspoon of salt per cup of flour.

Beware of baking powder, as well – one teaspoon could pack almost 500 milligrams of sodium. Most cake recipes need only a teaspoon of baking powder per cup of flour; muffins, biscuits, and waffles take a minimum of one and one-fourth teaspoons per cup of flour.

Hold the sugar. For yeast breads, try just one tablespoon of sugar per each cup of flour. Cakes can make do with even less – one-half cup of sugar per cup of flour. Pump up the flavor with vanilla, instead.

These are just a few hints to help you meet your meal plan and weight-loss goals. You'll find many more tips in the chapter *Proven plans from diet pros.*

Caramelized Garlic Chicken

2 teaspoons olive oil
4 garlic cloves, minced
4 teaspoons brown sugar
4 boneless, skinless chicken breast halves

☆ Heat oven to 500 degrees.
☆ Line shallow roasting pan with foil; spray foil with non-stick cooking spray.
☆ Heat oil in small nonstick skillet over medium-low heat until hot.
☆ Add garlic; cook 1 to 2 minutes or until garlic begins to soften, stirring frequently.
☆ Remove from heat; stir in brown sugar until well mixed.
☆ Place chicken breast halves in sprayed, foil-lined pan.
☆ Spread garlic mixture evenly over chicken.
☆ Bake at 500 degrees for 10 to 15 minutes or until chicken is fork-tender and juices run clear.

Serves 4. Per serving: 170 calories; 5g total fat; 5g carbohydrate; 27g protein; 75mg cholesterol; 65mg sodium; 5g sugars

Betty Crocker® Cookbook, 9th Edition, Betty Crocker website
Reprinted with permission of General Mills, Inc.

Chicken Diablo

1 package (about 1 pound) PERDUE® FIT 'N EASY®
Fresh Skinless & Boneless Chicken Breasts
2 tablespoons fresh lemon juice
1 tablespoon olive oil
2 garlic cloves, crushed
1/2 to 3/4 teaspoon crushed red pepper
1/2 to 3/4 teaspoon ground black pepper
Salt (optional)
1 lemon, sliced

☆ In shallow bowl, combine lemon juice, oil, garlic, peppers, and salt.

☆ Add chicken to marinade, turning to coat both sides. Cover and marinate in refrigerator 1 hour or longer.

☆ Preheat broiler.

☆ Drain chicken, reserving marinade.

☆ Broil 6 to 8 inches from heat source 6 to 8 minutes on each side until cooked through.

☆ Meanwhile, in a small saucepan, bring marinade to a boil.

☆ Turn chicken 2 or 3 times during cooking and brush with boiled marinade.

☆ To serve, garnish with lemon slices.

Serves 4. Per serving: 166 calories; 4.9g total fat; 4.3g carbohydrate; 26.7g protein; 1.5g dietary fiber; 113.79mg sodium

Light Sour Cream Chicken Enchiladas

1 (8-ounce) container light sour cream

1 (8-ounce) container nonfat plain yogurt

1 (10 3/4-ounce) can condensed, 99 percent fat-free cream of chicken soup with 1/3 less salt

1 (4-ounce) can diced green chiles

12 (6- or 7-inch) white corn or flour tortillas

4 ounces (1 cup) shredded cheddar cheese with 1/3 less fat

1 1/2 cups chopped cooked chicken

1/4 cup sliced green onions

☆ Heat oven to 350 degrees. Spray 13x9-inch (3-quart) baking dish with nonstick cooking spray.

☆ In medium bowl, combine sour cream, yogurt, soup, and chiles; mix well.

☆ Spoon about 3 tablespoons sour cream mixture down center of each tortilla.

☆ Reserve 1/4 cup of the cheese; sprinkle tortillas with remaining cheese, chicken, and onions.

☆ Roll up; place in sprayed dish. Spoon remaining sour cream mixture over tortillas. Cover with foil.

☆ Bake at 350 degrees for 25 to 30 minutes or until hot and bubbly.

☆ Remove foil; sprinkle with reserved 1/4 cup cheese. Bake uncovered for an additional 5 minutes or until cheese is melted.

☆ If desired, garnish with shredded lettuce and chopped tomatoes.

Serves 6. Per serving (2 tortillas): 350 calories; 11g total fat; 38g carbohydrate; 24g protein; 55mg cholesterol; 3g dietary fiber; 740mg sodium; 9g sugars

Betty Crocker® Cookbook, 9th Edition, Betty Crocker website
Reprinted with permission of General Mills, Inc.

Grilled Greek Chicken With Onions & Tomatoes

1 container (8 ounces) plain low-fat yogurt

2 cloves garlic, finely chopped

4 tablespoons olive or vegetable oil, divided

2 tablespoons chopped fresh mint and/or oregano

2 tablespoons lemon juice

1 tablespoon hot pepper sauce

1/2 teaspoon salt

1 package (1 1/4 pounds) PERDUE® FIT 'N EASY® Fresh Skinless & Boneless Chicken Breasts

2 onions, cut into wedges

1 tomato, seeded and coarsely chopped

☆ In large, shallow, non-aluminum baking dish, combine yogurt, garlic, 2 tablespoons oil, mint, oregano, lemon juice, hot pepper sauce, and salt until well-blended.

☆ Add chicken, turning to coat with marinade.

☆ Cover and marinate in refrigerator up to 3 hours.

☆ Preheat grill or broiler.

☆ In medium bowl, combine onions, remaining 2 tablespoons oil, and salt to taste and toss until evenly coated.

☆ Remove chicken from marinade and discard marinade.

☆ Grill or broil chicken, turning occasionally, 15 minutes or until meat thermometer inserted in center registers 170 degrees.

(continued on next page)

(continued)

☆ Grill onions in grill wok or on grill screen, stirring occasionally, until tender.

☆ Add tomato and grill just until heated through.

☆ Serve grilled vegetables over chicken.

Serves 4. Per serving: 346 calories; 16.4g total fat; 11.8g carbohydrate; 37g protein; 1.5g dietary fiber; 523.99mg sodium; 145.65mg calcium

Chicken McIntosh

1 cup New York State McIntosh apples cubed,
 unpeeled
2 cups cooked diced chicken
3/4 cup chopped peanuts
2 cans (10 1/2 ounces) chicken gravy
3 cups cooked buttered rice

☆ Combine chicken and gravy; heat in pan.
☆ Meanwhile, combine hot cooked rice and peanuts.
☆ Just before serving, add the cubed apples to the
  chicken, stir, and serve with the peanut rice.

Serves 4. Per serving: 615 calories; 27.6g total fat;
57.8g carbohydrate; 35.1g protein; 4.3g dietary fiber;
1028.83mg sodium

Chicken Sauté with Balsamic-Dried Plum Sauce

2 tablespoons olive oil

4 boneless, skinless chicken breast halves (about 1 1/2 pounds)

Salt and pepper

1/2 cup finely chopped shallots

2 cloves garlic, minced

1 cup chicken broth

1/2 cup (3 ounces) coarsely chopped dried plums

1/3 cup balsamic vinegar

1/2 teaspoon dried thyme leaves, crushed

☆ In large skillet, heat oil over medium heat until hot.

☆ Season chicken with salt and pepper, as desired.

☆ Place chicken in skillet; cook 10 minutes or until browned and centers are no longer pink, turning once.

☆ Transfer to serving platter; keep warm.

☆ Add shallots and garlic to same skillet; cook and stir 3 to 5 minutes or until softened.

☆ Stir in broth, dried plums, vinegar, thyme, 1/2 teaspoon salt, and 1/4 teaspoon pepper.

☆ Bring to a boil over high heat. Reduce heat slightly; cook until sauce is reduced by half, about 1 cup.

☆ Spoon over chicken.

Serves 4. Per serving: 330 calories; 9g total fat; 20g carbohydrate; 41g protein; 100mg cholesterol; 2g dietary fiber; 890mg sodium

Reprinted with permission from the California Dried Plum Board.

Vegetable Wraps with Chicken and Hummus

1 cup diced cooked chicken
1/2 cup chopped cucumber
1/2 cup chopped red bell pepper
1/2 cup chopped raw sugar snap peas
1/2 cup chopped arugula
1/2 cup hummus
4 wraps or flour tortillas
4 lettuce leaves (leaf or butter lettuce works best)

☆ Combine the chicken, cucumber, bell pepper, peas, arugula, and hummus in a bowl. (You can add different vegetables according to the season and your family's preferences.)

☆ Lay the wraps on the counter and cover each with a lettuce leaf.

☆ Divide the vegetable mixture among them and spread, leaving at least a 1/2-inch border around the edge.

☆ Roll up tightly, tucking in the edges as you roll.

☆ Cut in half and wrap in plastic food film.

Serves 4. Per serving: 190 calories; 3g total fat; 25g carbohydrate; 10g dietary fiber; 355mg sodium

Chicken Zorba

1 package (about 1 pound) PERDUE® FIT 'N EASY®
Fresh Thin-Sliced Skinless and Boneless Chicken
Breast Cutlets

1 teaspoon dried oregano leaves

Salt and ground pepper to taste

1 tablespoon olive oil

3 garlic cloves, crushed

1 can (14 1/2 ounces) Italian-style tomatoes

1/2 teaspoon fennel seed

8 ounces orzo pasta, cooked and drained

1/2 cup crumbled feta cheese

Freshly chopped parsley

1/3 cup Kalamata olives or other oil-cured black
olives (optional)

☆ Season breasts with oregano, salt, and pepper

☆ In large nonstick skillet, over medium-high heat,
heat oil.

☆ Add garlic; sauté 2 minutes and remove.

☆ Add chicken and brown 1 1/2 to 2 1/2 minutes per
side. Stir in tomatoes and fennel seed.

☆ Reduce heat to medium-low and simmer, uncovered,
5 minutes to blend flavors.

☆ Serve chicken and sauce over pasta.

☆ Sprinkle with feta and parsley and garnish with olives.

Serves 4. Per serving: 312 calories; 10.5g total fat; 20.9g
carbohydrate; 32.4g protein; 2g dietary fiber; 492.28mg
sodium; 149.45mg calcium

Slow-Cooked White Chili With Chicken

1 pound boneless, skinless chicken thighs, cut into thin strips

1 cup dried great northern beans, rinsed, sorted

1 medium onion, chopped

1 garlic clove, minced

2 teaspoons dried oregano leaves

1/2 teaspoon salt

1 (10 3/4-ounce) can condensed cream of chicken soup

5 cups water

1 teaspoon cumin

1/4 teaspoon hot pepper sauce

1 (4 1/2-ounce) can of Old El Paso® Chopped Green Chiles

Fresh sage, if desired

☆ In 3 1/2- or 4-quart slow cooker, combine chicken, beans, onion, garlic, oregano, salt, soup, and water; mix well.

☆ Cover; cook on low setting for 8 to 10 hours or until beans are tender and chicken is no longer pink.

☆ Just before serving, stir in cumin, hot pepper sauce, and chiles.

☆ Serve with additional hot sauce if desired. Garnish with sage.

Serves 6. Per serving (1 1/2 cups): 260 calories; 9g total fat; 23g carbohydrate; 21g protein; 50mg cholesterol; 6g dietary fiber; 700mg sodium; 2g sugars

Betty Crocker® Cookbook, 9th Edition, Betty Crocker website
Reprinted with permission of General Mills, Inc.

Chicken Bulgur Salad

1 package (about 1 pound) PERDUE® FIT 'N
EASY® Fresh Skinless and Boneless Chicken
Breast Tenderloins
1 cup bulgur wheat
2 tomatoes, peeled, seeded, and chopped
1/4 cup fresh basil leaves
2 tablespoons extra virgin olive oil
2 tablespoons red wine vinegar
1 garlic clove, minced
1 tablespoon chopped fresh mint leaves
Salt and pepper to taste
1 head Romaine lettuce, separated into leaves
1/2 cup minced fresh parsley (optional)

☆ Prepare bulgur according to package directions.
☆ Meanwhile, in large saucepan or skillet over high heat,
   bring 2 inches water to boil.
☆ Add chicken tenderloins.
☆ Reduce heat to medium-low. Cover and poach 7 to 10
   minutes until cooked through.
☆ Let tenderloins cool in liquid about 10 minutes.
☆ Shred chicken into bite-sized pieces.
☆ In medium-sized bowl, toss bulgur with chicken, toma-
   toes, basil, oil, vinegar, garlic, and mint; season with
   salt and pepper.
☆ To serve, mound salad on bed of Romaine lettuce;
   garnish with parsley.

Serves 4. Per serving: 329 calories; 9g total fat;
31.8g carbohydrate; 31.9g protein; 8g dietary fiber;
130.94mg sodium

Summer Fruit and Chicken Salad

Dressing:
1/2 cup low-fat raspberry yogurt
1/4 cup light mayonnaise or salad dressing
2 tablespoons honey

Salad:
4 leaves leaf lettuce
8 ounces sliced, cooked chicken, cut into bite-
    sized strips
1/2 medium cantaloupe, seeds removed, peeled, cut
    into very thin slices, and halved
1 cup fresh raspberries
1/2 cup fresh blueberries

☆ In small bowl, combine all dressing ingredients; blend
  well. Refrigerate until serving time.
☆ To serve, arrange lettuce on large serving platter or on
  4 individual plates.
☆ Arrange chicken, cantaloupe, raspberries, and blueberries over lettuce.
☆ Drizzle dressing over salad.

Serves 4. Per serving: 290 calories; 10g total fat; 31g carbohydrate; 20g protein; 55mg cholesterol; 190mg
sodium; 26g sugars

Betty Crocker® Cookbook, 9th Edition, Betty Crocker website
Reprinted with permission of General Mills, Inc.

Summer Salad Sandwich

2 cups watermelon wedges, seeded
1 cup cooked chicken, chopped
1 tablespoon chopped cilantro
2 tablespoons plain low-fat yogurt
1/4 teaspoon garlic salt
1/8 teaspoon cayenne pepper
2 pita breads, halved
1/4 cup low-fat cream cheese
4 large lettuce leaves

☆ Place cubed watermelon on paper towels to remove excess liquid.

☆ Mix chicken, cilantro, yogurt, garlic salt, and cayenne pepper.

☆ Spread inside surface of pita bread halves with herb cheese and fill each with about 1/4 cup chicken mixture.

☆ Arrange watermelon and lettuce in pita bread.

Serves 4. Per serving (1/2 pita): 190 calories; 3g total fat; 24g carbohydrate; 16g protein; 1g dietary fiber; 305mg sodium

Heart-Healthful Turkey Reubens

1/4 cup nonfat Thousand Island salad dressing
8 slices dark rye or pumpernickel bread
8 ounces thinly sliced, low-fat, low-sodium cooked
    turkey or chicken
1/2 cup sauerkraut, rinsed and well drained
4 slices low-fat Swiss cheese (1 1/2 ounces)
Vegetable oil spray

☆ Spread salad dressing on one side of each slice
   of bread.
☆ Top 4 slices of bread with turkey or chicken,
   sauerkraut, and cheese.
☆ Top with remaining bread slices, dressing side down.
☆ Spray a large skillet with vegetable oil.
☆ Cook 2 sandwiches over medium heat for 4 to 6
   minutes, or until bread toasts and cheese melts,
   turning once.
☆ Repeat with remaining sandwiches.

Serves 4. Per serving: 273 calories; 5g total fat; 31g carbohydrate; 24g protein; 48mg cholesterol; 780mg sodium

Skillet Chili

1/2 jalapeño chili or 2 tablespoons canned jalapeño chili slices, mild, chopped

1 tablespoon vegetable oil

1 1/2 cups chopped onion

1 1/2 cups chopped red bell pepper or 1 cup canned roasted red peppers

1 clove garlic, minced

1 1/2 to 3 teaspoons chili powder

1 teaspoon cumin

1/2 teaspoon salt

1 can (28 ounces) tomato purée with tomato bits

1 can (15 1/2 ounces) light red kidney beans

1 to 2 cups chopped, cooked Butterball® Boneless Young Turkey

☆ Trim, seed, and finely chop 1/2 jalapeño chili if using fresh chili pepper.

☆ Heat oil in skillet. Add onion, red bell pepper, jalapeño chili, garlic, chili powder, cumin, and salt.

☆ Sauté 4 to 5 minutes.

☆ Add tomato purée and beans, including liquid from can. Stir in turkey.

☆ Simmer for 5 minutes more.

Serves 7. Per serving (1 cup): 160 calories; 11g total fat; 820mg sodium

Velvet Turkey and Herbs

1 pound turkey breast tenderloins or boneless, skinless chicken breasts, all visible fat removed

Vegetable oil spray

1/4 cup chopped shallots or onion

1/2 teaspoon bottled minced garlic

2 tablespoons all-purpose flour

1 1/4 cups evaporated skim milk

1 tablespoon snipped fresh oregano or 1/2 teaspoon dried oregano, crushed

1 tablespoon snipped fresh parsley

1 teaspoon snipped fresh basil or 1/4 teaspoon dried basil, crushed

☆ Rinse turkey or chicken and pat dry. Cut into bite-sized pieces.

☆ Spray a skillet with vegetable oil. Place over medium-high heat.

☆ Add turkey or chicken, shallots or onion, and garlic to hot skillet. Cook 3 to 4 minutes, or until turkey or chicken is tender and no longer pink.

☆ Stir flour into mixture in skillet. Add remaining ingredients. Cook and stir until thickened and bubbly, about 3 minutes.

☆ Cook 1 minute more, stirring constantly.

Serves 4. Per serving (2/3 cup): 225 calories; 4g total fat; 13g carbohydrate; 33g protein; 70mg cholesterol; 155mg sodium

Zesty Turkey Wrap

2 cups finely chopped, cooked Butterball® Turkey
1/4 cup sliced green onions
1/4 cup finely chopped sun-dried tomatoes
1/2 cup prepared ranch salad dressing
Lettuce leaves
6 (7-inch diameter) flour tortillas or 4 pita pockets

☆ Combine turkey, onions, tomatoes, and dressing in medium bowl.
☆ Place lettuce leaves toward one edge of each tortilla.
☆ Divide turkey salad among tortillas, placing on lettuce.
☆ Roll to wrap.
☆ If using pita pockets, cut pockets in half, line with lettuce, and add turkey salad.

Serves 6. Per serving: 340 calories; 15.5g total fat; 30g carbohydrate; 19g protein; 2.3g dietary fiber; 504.19mg sodium

Ginger Sesame Salmon

4 sheets (12x18 inches each) Reynolds Wrap® Everyday® Heavy Duty Aluminum Foil

4 thin onion slices, separated in rings

2 medium carrots, cut in julienne strips or shredded

4 salmon fillets (4 to 6 ounces each), thawed

2 teaspoons grated fresh ginger

2 tablespoons seasoned rice vinegar

1 teaspoon sesame oil

Salt and pepper

Fresh spinach leaves

☆ Preheat oven to 450 degrees or grill to medium-high.

☆ Center onions and carrots on each sheet of Reynolds Wrap® Everyday® Heavy Duty Aluminum Foil.

☆ Top with salmon. Sprinkle with ginger; drizzle with vinegar and oil. Sprinkle with salt and pepper.

☆ Bring up foil sides. Double-fold top and ends to seal packet, leaving room for heat circulation inside. Repeat to make 4 packets.

☆ Bake 16 to 20 minutes on a cookie sheet in oven, or grill 14 to 18 minutes in covered grill.

☆ Serve salmon and vegetables on a bed of spinach. Sprinkle with additional seasoned rice vinegar, if desired.

Serves 4. Per serving: 378 calories; 16g total fat; 9g carbohydrate; 47g protein; 101mg cholesterol; 723mg sodium

Reprinted with permission from The Reynolds Kitchens.

Marinated Mediterranean-style Alaska Salmon Steaks

6 ounces frozen limeade, thawed

3/4 cup olive oil

3/4 cup soy sauce

2 tablespoons minced fresh garlic

2 tablespoons chopped fresh rosemary

6 (4 to 6 ounces each) Alaska salmon, halibut, or cod steaks/fillets*

☆ Combine limeade, olive oil, soy sauce, garlic, and rosemary in a shallow baking dish.

☆ Place seafood in dish. Turn fish over several times to coat; refrigerate 30 to 45 minutes.

☆ Remove seafood from marinade.

☆ Cook seafood on oiled, medium-hot grill, turning once during cooking, about 6 to 12 minutes per inch of thickness. Do not overcook.

Serves 6. Per serving: 530 calories; 33g total fat; 21g carbohydrate; 38g protein; 0.6g dietary fiber; 2125.49mg sodium

*If using Alaska halibut or cod, substitute 1 teaspoon each of dried oregano and ground coriander for rosemary. Proceed as directed.

Poached Salmon with Spinach

1 pound salmon fillets

1 1/2 cups water

1/2 cup dry white wine or water

2 green onions, sliced

1 bay leaf

1/2 of a 10-ounce package frozen, no-salt-added, chopped spinach

1/8 teaspoon ground nutmeg

1/4 cup shredded part-skim mozzarella cheese

Freshly ground black pepper

Lemon slices (optional)

☆ Cut salmon into 4 pieces, rinse, and pat dry. Set aside.

☆ In a large skillet, combine water, wine, green onions, and bay leaf. Over high heat, bring just to a boil.

☆ Carefully add salmon and return to a boil.

☆ Reduce heat, cover, and simmer 8 to 10 minutes or until fish flakes easily with a fork.

☆ Remove fish and pat it dry with paper towels.

☆ Cut each salmon steak in half, removing as much of the bone, cartilage, and skin as possible.

☆ Meanwhile, cook spinach according to package directions. Drain well, squeezing out moisture. Stir in nutmeg.

☆ Preheat broiler.

☆ Place fish on a broiler-proof serving platter or on the rack of an unheated broiler pan.

(continued on next page)

(continued)

☆ Top with spinach mixture, sprinkle with cheese, and season with pepper.

☆ Broil 4 inches from the heat for 1 to 2 minutes or until cheese melts.

☆ Garnish with lemon slices, if desired.

Serves 4. Per serving: 190 calories; 8g total fat; 2g carbohydrate; 27g protein; 47mg cholesterol; 110mg sodium

Salmon with Yogurt Herb Sauce

4 sheets (12x18 inches each) Reynolds Wrap® Every-
day® Heavy Duty Aluminum Foil

Nonstick olive oil cooking spray

4 salmon fillets (4 to 6 ounces each)

Salt and pepper to taste

1 medium cucumber, peeled, seeded, and cut into
1/2-inch cubes (to make 1 1/2 cups)

1 tablespoon chopped fresh dill or 1 teaspoon dried
dill weed

Sauce:

1 cup plain low-fat yogurt

1 tablespoon chopped fresh dill or 1 teaspoon dried
dill weed

1 tablespoon chopped parsley

1 tablespoon olive oil

2 teaspoons Dijon mustard

1/2 teaspoon sugar

Salt and pepper

☆ Preheat oven to 450 degrees or preheat grill to
medium-high.

☆ Spray foil with nonstick, olive oil cooking spray.

☆ Center one salmon fillet on each sheet of Reynolds
Wrap® Everyday® Heavy Duty Aluminum Foil.

☆ Sprinkle with salt and pepper. Top with cucumber
and dill.

(continued on next page)

(continued)

☆ Bring up foil sides. Double-fold top and ends to seal packet, leaving room for heat circulation inside. Repeat to make 4 packets.

☆ Bake 10 to 14 minutes on a cookie sheet in oven, or grill 8 to 12 minutes in covered grill.

☆ Combine yogurt, dill, parsley, olive oil, mustard, sugar, salt, and pepper. Serve with salmon.

☆ Garnish with fresh dill, if desired.

Serves 4. Per serving: 277 calories; 10g total fat; 7g carbohydrate; 37g protein; 92mg cholesterol; 801mg sodium

Reprinted with permission from The Reynolds Kitchens.

Crispy Baked Filet of Sole

1 1/2 pounds sole fillets
3/4 cup finely chopped onion
1/2 cup acceptable vegetable oil
1/4 cup fresh lime juice
2 teaspoons grated lime rind
1 tablespoon grated fresh ginger
1 tablespoon light soy sauce
1/4 teaspoon salt
1/4 teaspoon ground white pepper
Vegetable oil spray
1 1/4 cups plain bread crumbs
2 tablespoons finely chopped fresh parsley
2 tablespoons finely chopped green onion

☆ Rinse fish and pat dry. Set aside.

☆ In a small bowl, combine onion, oil, lime juice and rind, ginger, soy sauce, salt, and pepper. Set aside.

☆ Lay fillets in a baking dish and pour liquid mixture over all, turning fillets to coat evenly. Cover and refrigerate for several hours or overnight.

☆ Preheat oven to 450 degrees. Lightly spray a baking dish with vegetable oil spray.

☆ In a pie plate, combine bread crumbs, parsley, and green onion. Stir to mix well, and set aside.

☆ Remove fillets from marinade and coat with crumb mixture. Place fillets in prepared baking dish and bake 15 to 18 minutes or until fish flakes easily with a fork.

Serves 6. Per serving: 339 calories; 20g total fat; 17g carbohydrate; 22g protein; 54mg cholesterol; 427mg sodium

Easy Meatloaf

1 1/2 pounds lean ground beef

1 cup tomato sauce, catsup, or barbecue (BBQ) sauce

1 1/4 cups Quaker® Oats, (quick or old-fashioned variety, uncooked)

1 large egg or 2 egg whites, lightly beaten

1/4 cup chopped onion

1/2 teaspoon salt (optional)

1/4 teaspoon pepper

☆ Heat oven to 350 degrees.

☆ Combine all ingredients; mix lightly but thoroughly.

☆ Pat into 8x4-inch loaf pan.

☆ Bake 1 hour or until meat is no longer pink and juices run clear.

☆ Let meatloaf stand for 5 minutes before cutting. Drain off any juices before slicing.

Serves 8. Per serving: 340 calories; 20g total fat; 18.9g carbohydrate; 20.4g protein; 3.1g dietary fiber; 397.85mg sodium

Barley Lentil Soup

2 to 3 cloves garlic, finely chopped
1 cup chopped onion
2 medium carrots, peeled and chopped
1 stalk celery, chopped
7 cups salt-reduced, fat-free chicken broth, divided
1 1/2 cups small, fresh button mushrooms, sliced
1 cup lentils, rinsed
1/2 cup pearl barley
1 tablespoon tomato paste
1 1/2 teaspoons dried leaf thyme, crushed
1 teaspoon curry powder
1 bay leaf
1 tablespoon finely chopped Italian parsley
2 tablespoons fresh lemon juice
1 tablespoon Worcestershire sauce
1 teaspoon salt
1/2 teaspoon ground black pepper

- ☆ Spray 4-quart saucepan with nonstick cooking spray.
- ☆ Add onion and garlic; sauté 4 minutes, stirring occasionally. Add carrots and celery; sauté 3 minutes longer, stirring occasionally.
- ☆ Mix in 6 cups broth, mushrooms, lentils, barley, tomato paste, thyme, curry powder, and bay leaf.
- ☆ Bring to a boil.

(continued on next page)

(continued)

☆ Reduce heat and simmer 60 to 70 minutes or until lentils and barley are tender but not mushy.

☆ Blend in remaining broth, lemon juice, Worcestershire sauce, salt, and pepper.

☆ Remove bay leaf and serve.

Serves 8. Per serving: 186 calories; 4g total fat; 31g carbohydrate; 10g protein; 10g dietary fiber; 4mg cholesterol; 1092mg sodium

© Barley Lentil Soup
Reprinted with permission from the National Barley Foods Council.

Pasta with Sweet Potato Sauce

1 pound sweet potatoes, about 3 medium
1/8 teaspoon salt
1/2 pound cooked pasta
2 tablespoons chopped parsley
1 12-ounce can evaporated skim milk
1/4 teaspoon ground white pepper
4 tablespoons grated Parmesan cheese
Pasta of choice

☆ Peel and slice sweet potatoes and steam for about 14 minutes until soft.

☆ Place cooked potatoes into blender with milk and whisk for about 7 minutes. The mixture will become a glossy, rich color.

☆ Season with salt and pepper and pour over cooked pasta.

☆ Sprinkle with grated Parmesan cheese and parsley.

Serves 4. Per serving: 250 calories; 2.2g total fat; 44.9g carbohydrate; 12.7g protein; 3.6g dietary fiber; 289.9mg sodium; 372.8mg calcium

Open-Face Vegetable Sandwiches

2 to 4 teaspoons Dijon mustard
2 whole-grain English muffins, split and toasted
1/2 cup small broccoli florets
1/4 cup chopped red, yellow, or green bell pepper
1/4 cup shredded carrot
1/2 cup shredded, low-fat Monterey Jack cheese

☆ Preheat broiler.

☆ Spread mustard over the cut side of each English muffin half.

☆ Arrange broccoli, bell pepper, and carrot over mustard. Sprinkle with cheese.

☆ Place English muffin halves on the unheated rack of a broiler pan.

☆ Broil about 4 inches from the heat for 2 to 3 minutes or until cheese melts.

Serves 2. Per serving: 246 calories; 6g total fat; 34g carbohydrate; 14g protein; 17mg cholesterol; 352mg sodium

Reproduced with permission
Recipes
© 2003, Copyright American Heart Association

Vegetable Burritos

1 teaspoon olive oil
1 sweet onion (2 cups)
3 cloves garlic
1 red bell pepper (1 cup)
2 cups sliced mushrooms
1/2 teaspoon cumin
1 teaspoon chili powder
Dash of salt
1 can (15 ounces) of reduced-sodium black beans
    (1 1/2 cups)
4 flour tortillas
1/2 cup chopped cilantro

☆ Preheat the oven to 350 degrees.

☆ Heat the oil in a high-sided skillet. Sauté the onions until soft and just slightly golden, 5 minutes.

☆ Add the garlic, bell pepper, and mushrooms and cook until the vegetables are tender, about 5 minutes.

☆ Stir in the black beans with a little of their liquid and heat through.

☆ Heat the tortillas in a paper bag in the microwave about 1 minute.

☆ Lay the warm tortillas on the counter, divide the filling among them, and scatter cilantro on top. Roll, turning in the sides, into a neat package.

☆ Lay in a baking dish covered lightly with aluminum foil and warm through in the oven, 10 minutes (20 to 30 minutes if they have been made earlier and chilled).

Serves 6. Per serving: 231 calories; 5g total fat; 44g carbohydrate; 9g dietary fiber; 362mg sodium

Recipes:
slimming side dishes

California Cucumber Salad

2 cucumbers, scrubbed, not peeled
1/3 cup raisins
1/4 cup chopped, unsalted, dry-roasted walnuts
1/4 cup plain nonfat yogurt

☆ Shred cucumbers and drain.
☆ Place in a medium bowl and add remaining ingredients. Toss to mix well.
☆ Serve on lettuce-lined salad plates.

Serves 4. Per serving: 109 calories; 5g total fat; 16g carbohydrate; 3g protein; 0mg cholesterol; 18mg sodium

Citrus Slaw

1/4 cup prepared nonfat herb vinaigrette
1/4 cup frozen orange juice concentrate, thawed
4 cups shredded napa cabbage
2 oranges, peeled and segmented
1 red apple, halved, cored, and diced
1 cup (about 6 ounces) pitted dried plums, quartered
1/2 cup sliced celery
1/4 cup sliced green onions
Pepper (optional)

☆ In large bowl, whisk together vinaigrette and juice concentrate.
☆ Add cabbage, oranges, apple, dried plums, celery, and green onions, tossing to coat.
☆ Season with pepper, if desired.

Serves 6. Per serving: 113 calories; 0g total fat; 28g carbohydrate; 2g protein; 0mg cholesterol; 6g dietary fiber; 155mg sodium

Reprinted with permission from the California Dried Plum Board.

Classic Waldorf Salad

2 cups diced, unpared New York State apples (about
   2 medium apples)

1 cup diced celery

1/3 cup coarsely chopped walnuts

1/2 cup mayonnaise*

☆ Combine apple, celery, nuts, and mayonnaise; toss.

☆ If desired, mound salad in lettuce cups to serve.

*Mayonnaise substitutes:

1/4 cup plain (or vanilla) yogurt

1/4 cup mayonnaise

Or

1/2 cup plain (or vanilla) yogurt

1 tablespoon maple syrup

Serves 4 to 6. Per serving (with mayonnaise): 308 calories; 28.6g total fat; 13.7g carbohydrate; 2.2g protein; 3g
dietary fiber; 182.61mg sodium

Per serving (with maple syrup): 143 calories; 7.3g total fat;
18.5g carbohydrate; 3.5g protein; 3g dietary fiber;
48.25mg sodium

Reprinted with permission from the New York Apple Association.

Get-to-Know-Your-Greens Salad

1 8-ounce can citrus salad in its own juice
1 8-ounce can apricot halves in its own juice
1 teaspoon extra virgin olive oil
4 teaspoons raspberry or white wine vinegar
1/4 teaspoon salt
1/4 teaspoon black pepper
2 cups bite-sized pieces of endive
1 cup bite-sized pieces of arugula
1 cup bite-sized pieces of watercress

☆ Drain citrus salad and apricots and reserve liquid in a small bowl.

☆ Slice apricot halves lengthwise into four slices each. Set fruit aside.

☆ Whisk together canning liquid, olive oil, vinegar, salt, and pepper.

☆ Combine greens in a large salad bowl. Add fruit and dressing and toss. Serve.

Serves 4. Per serving: 86 calories; 1.2g total fat; 18g carbohydrate; 1g protein; 0mg cholesterol; 2g dietary fiber; 156mg sodium

Romaine Salad with Orange Vinaigrette

1 Reynolds® Pot Lux™ Cookware, 1 1/2-quart pan

Salad:

1/2 package (10 ounces) fresh Romaine lettuce
   leaves (4 cups)
1/2 cup matchstick carrots
1/2 medium red delicious apple, cut in large chunks
1/2 cup seedless red grapes
1/2 cup mandarin oranges, drained
1/4 cup pecan pieces

Orange Vinaigrette:

1/4 cup sweet orange marmalade
2 tablespoons white wine vinegar
1 tablespoon olive oil
1/8 teaspoon ground ginger

☆ Place first 4 salad ingredients in Pot Lux™ pan;
   toss gently.
☆ Arrange oranges on top of salad mixture. Cover and
   refrigerate until serving time.
☆ Combine all ingredients for Orange Vinaigrette;
   set aside.
☆ Drizzle with Orange Vinaigrette, top with pecans, and
   toss gently before serving.

Serves 6 to 8. Per serving: 244 calories, 9g fat; 43g carbohydrate; 2g protein; 0mg cholesterol; 4g dietary fiber;
33mg sodium

Reprinted with permission from The Reynolds Kitchens.

Tangy Apple Salad

3 New York State Empire apples
4 heads Boston or Bibb lettuce (or 1 head
  Romaine lettuce)
2/3 cup plain low-fat yogurt
1 tablespoon orange marmalade
Freshly ground black pepper to taste
1/4 cup sliced almonds

☆ Mix yogurt with marmalade and pepper.
☆ Tear lettuce into bite-size pieces.
☆ Cut apples into small cubes.
☆ Mix lettuce, apples, almonds, and dressing.
☆ Serve immediately.

Serves 5. Per serving: 116 calories; 3.1g total fat; 1.9mg
cholesterol; 2.9g dietary fiber; 30mg sodium

Reprinted with permission from the New York Apple Association.

Asparagus with Mustard Sauce

1 sheet (18x24 inches) Reynolds Wrap® Heavy Duty
Aluminum Foil
2 pounds asparagus, trimmed
3 tablespoons margarine or butter
Salt and pepper

Sauce:
1 cup light sour cream
2 tablespoons red wine vinegar
1/4 cup Dijon mustard
2 teaspoons sugar
1/8 teaspoon crushed red pepper

☆ Preheat oven to 450 degrees or grill to medium-high.
☆ Center asparagus on sheet of Reynolds Wrap®
   Heavy Duty Aluminum Foil; top with margarine.
☆ Bring up foil sides. Double-fold top and ends to
   seal, making 1 large foil packet, leaving room for
   heat circulation inside.
☆ Bake 14 to 16 minutes on a cookie sheet in oven, or
   grill 7 to 9 minutes in covered grill.
☆ Open foil; season with salt and pepper.
☆ Combine sour cream, vinegar, mustard, sugar, and red
   pepper in small, microwave-safe bowl to make sauce.
☆ Microwave on high power 1 1/2 to 2 minutes or until
   warm. Serve sauce over asparagus.

Serves 6 to 8. Per serving: 114 calories; 6g total fat; 12g
carbohydrate; 4g protein; 21mg cholesterol; 2g dietary
fiber; 402mg sodium

Reprinted with permission from The Reynolds Kitchens.

Braised Chestnuts

2 cups canned chestnuts, drained (be sure they are
    not in a sugar syrup)
1 cup low-sodium chicken broth or dry red wine
1/4 teaspoon dried thyme
1/4 teaspoon dried sage
2 teaspoons cornstarch mixed with 2 tablespoons
    water (slurry)
1 tablespoon freshly chopped, or 1 teaspoon
    dried, parsley

☆ Simmer the chestnuts in the broth or wine with the
    thyme and sage 20 minutes.
☆ Stir in the slurry and stir to thicken and clear.
☆ Add the parsley and serve with a holiday bird or
    other roast.

Serves 4. Per serving: 148 calories; 1g total fat; 33g carbohydrate; 0g dietary fiber; 157mg sodium

Glazed Carrots with Dried Plums

1 pound (6 medium) carrots, peeled and cut into
   2-inch pieces or baby carrots
1/2 cup orange juice
1 tablespoon honey
2 teaspoons prepared yellow mustard
1/8 teaspoon pepper
1 cup (about 6 ounces) pitted dried plums, halved
1 tablespoon butter
Salt to taste
2 tablespoons chopped parsley (optional)

☆ In large skillet, cover carrots with water. Bring to a boil.

☆ Reduce heat to medium. Cook about 10 minutes or
   until crisp-tender; drain and return to skillet.

☆ Meanwhile, in small bowl, whisk together orange juice,
   honey, mustard, and pepper; set aside.

☆ Add dried plums, butter, and orange juice mixture
   to carrots.

☆ Cover and cook over low heat 5 to 10 minutes or
   until sauce thickens slightly and is reduced by half,
   stirring occasionally.

☆ Season to taste with salt. Garnish with parsley,
   if desired.

Serves 6. Per serving: 156 calories; 2g total fat; 33g carbohydrate; 2g protein; 5mg cholesterol; 4g dietary fiber; 169mg sodium

Reprinted with permission from the California Dried Plum Board.

Greek Garden Vegetables

1 sheet (18x24 inches) Reynolds Wrap® Heavy Duty
   Aluminum Foil
4 cups broccoli florets
2 1/2 cups cauliflowerettes
1 pint cherry tomatoes
1/4 cup pitted, sliced kalamata olives or sliced
   ripe olives
1 1/2 teaspoons dried oregano
Salt and pepper
2 ice cubes
1/4 cup crumbled feta cheese

☆ Preheat oven to 450 degrees or grill to medium-high.
☆ Center broccoli, cauliflowerettes, tomatoes, and
   olives on sheet of Reynolds Wrap® Heavy Duty
   Aluminum Foil.
☆ Sprinkle with oregano, salt, and pepper. Top with
   ice cubes.
☆ Bring up foil sides. Double-fold top and ends to
   seal, making 1 large packet, leaving room for heat
   circulation inside.
☆ Bake 20 to 25 minutes on a cookie sheet in oven, or
   grill 12 to 14 minutes in covered grill.
☆ Sprinkle with feta cheese before serving.

Serves 4. Per serving: 105 calories; 4g total fat; 15g carbohydrate; 6g protein; 5mg cholesterol; 3g dietary fiber;
555mg sodium

Reprinted with permission from The Reynolds Kitchens.

Green Bean Almondine

1 pound fresh green beans (about 3 cups)
1 teaspoon light margarine
1/4 cup low-sodium vegetable or chicken broth
1 tablespoon chopped fresh oregano or 1 teaspoon
  dried, crumbled
Freshly ground pepper to taste
1 cup frozen pearl onions (about 4 ounces)
2 tablespoons sliced almonds
1/4 cup seasoned bread crumbs

☆ Trim green beans and slice into 2-inch sections.

☆ In a large nonstick skillet, heat margarine over medium-high heat.

☆ Add green beans and sauté 1 to 2 minutes, stirring constantly so beans cook evenly.

☆ Add broth, oregano, and pepper; sauté for 20 to 30 seconds. Add onions.

☆ Cook covered over medium-low heat for 6 to 8 minutes or until beans are tender-crisp.

☆ Meanwhile, in a small nonstick pan over medium heat, dry-roast almonds, stirring occasionally, for 2 to 3 minutes.

☆ Sprinkle bread crumbs and almonds over cooked beans.

Serves 6. Per serving: 61 calories; 1g total fat; 10g carbohydrate; 2g protein; 0mg cholesterol; 64mg sodium

Reproduced with permission
Recipes
© 2003, Copyright American Heart Association

Italian-Style Spaghetti Squash

1/2 medium spaghetti squash (about 1 1/2 pounds —
see note)

2 tablespoons water

14 1/2-ounce can Italian-style stewed tomatoes, drained

1/4 cup grated or shredded Parmesan cheese
(optional)

☆ Remove seeds from squash.

☆ Place squash cut-side down in a microwave-safe baking dish. Add water.

☆ Cover and microwave on 100 percent power (high)
for 10 to 14 minutes, or until pulp can just be
pierced with a fork; give dish a 1/2 turn twice during
cooking. Drain.

☆ Using pot holders, hold squash in one hand and with a
fork shred squash pulp into strands, letting them fall
into the baking dish.

☆ Add drained tomatoes, tossing to coat.

☆ Sprinkle with Parmesan cheese if desired.

Conventional Oven Cooking Method:

☆ Prepare recipe as above, except prick the squash skin
all over with a fork.

☆ Bake, uncovered, in a glass baking dish in a preheated
350-degree oven for 30 to 40 minutes or until tender.

☆ Complete recipe as above.

(continued on next page)

(continued)

Note:

★ Buy a 3-pound squash and cut it in half lengthwise.

★ Use one piece for this recipe and cover and refrigerate the other piece to try another time. The uncooked squash will stay fresh for up to 1 week.

Serves 6. Per serving (1/2 cup): 42 calories; 0g total fat; 9g carbohydrate; 1g protein; 0mg cholesterol; 112mg sodium

Mushroom Quesadillas

Vegetable oil spray

8 ounces sliced fresh mushrooms

1/2 medium onion, thinly sliced and separated
  into rings

1 teaspoon bottled minced garlic

3 tablespoons chopped fresh cilantro

3 8-inch whole-wheat flour tortillas

6 tablespoons shredded low-fat Monterey Jack
  cheese with jalapeño peppers, or low-fat
  cheddar cheese

Salsa (optional)

☆ Preheat oven to 350 degrees. Spray a large skillet
  with vegetable oil.

☆ Cook mushrooms, onion, and garlic in skillet over
  medium heat until onion is tender, about 5 to 7 minutes. Stir in cilantro and remove from heat.

☆ Arrange 1/3 of the mushroom mixture on half of 1 tortilla. Sprinkle with 2 tablespoons of the cheese.

☆ Fold the other half of the tortilla over cheese. Place on
  a baking sheet. Repeat with remaining ingredients to
  make 3 quesadillas total.

☆ Bake quesadillas about 5 minutes, or until filling is hot
  and cheese melts.

☆ Cut each quesadilla into 4 wedges. Serve warm with
  salsa if desired.

(continued on next page)

(continued)

Microwave Method:

☆ Spray a microwave-safe casserole with vegetable oil.

☆ Add mushrooms, onion, and garlic.

☆ Cook uncovered on 100 percent power (high) for 5 to 7 minutes or until onion is tender, stirring twice.

☆ Stir in cilantro.

☆ Assemble quesadillas as directed above and arrange them on a microwave-safe plate or platter.

☆ Cook, rotating plate once, uncovered on 100-percent power (high) for 1 to 2 minutes or until filling is hot and cheese melts.

Serves 6. Per serving (2 wedges): 67 calories; 2g total fat; 10g carbohydrate; 4g protein; 4mg cholesterol; 115mg sodium

Reproduced with permission
Recipes
© 2003, Copyright American Heart Association

Sweet Potato Casserole

4 medium sweet potatoes
Vegetable oil spray
1 tablespoon acceptable margarine
1/4 cup orange juice
2 tablespoons chopped walnuts
1/4 teaspoon nutmeg

☆ Cook whole sweet potatoes in boiling water 25 to 30 minutes or until tender.

☆ Meanwhile, preheat oven to 375 degrees.

☆ Lightly spray a 1-quart casserole dish with vegetable oil spray.

☆ Remove potatoes from heat and add cold water until potatoes are cooled slightly. Peel and mash.

☆ Add remaining ingredients and mix thoroughly.

☆ Place in casserole dish and bake uncovered 25 minutes. Serve hot.

Serves 6. Per serving: 116 calories; 4g total fat; 20g carbohydrate; 2g protein; 0mg cholesterol; 9mg sodium

Sweet Potato & Apple Casserole

3 medium New York State apples
3 medium sweet potatoes
1/4 teaspoon salt
1/4 cup sugar
1/2 teaspoon nutmeg
1 tablespoon grated orange peel
1/4 cup orange juice

☆ Wash and prick sweet potatoes with a fork and micro-wave on high for 8 minutes. Slip the skins and slice into 1/2-inch slices.

☆ Peel apples and slice crosswise into 1/2-inch rings.

☆ Combine salt, sugar, nutmeg, and orange peel in a small bowl.

☆ Alternate slices of sweet potatoes and apples in a deep 1 1/2-quart casserole dish.

☆ Sprinkle sugar mixture over each layer. Add orange juice and cover.

☆ Microwave on high for 6 minutes.

Serves 6. Per serving: 134 calories; 0g total fat; 0mg cholesterol; 3g dietary fiber; 95mg sodium

Reprinted with permission from the New York Apple Association.

Broiled Mixed Vegetables

1 2-pound package frozen mixed vegetables of your
   choice (6 cups)
2 teaspoons olive oil
1/4 teaspoon salt
1/4 teaspoon pepper
1/4 teaspoon rosemary

☆ Preheat the broiler. Place a rack with very small open
    squares on a broiler pan or baking sheet.

☆ Place the frozen vegetables, oil, salt, pepper, and
    rosemary in a plastic bag. Shake to coat the vegeta-
    bles with the oil and seasonings.

☆ Spread on the broiler rack. Broil 6 minutes, 4 inches
    from the heat source.

Serves 4 to 6. Per serving: 148 calories; 2g total fat; 23g
carbohydrate; 5g dietary fiber; 255mg sodium

Zucchini Tomato Vegetable Packet

1 sheet (18x24 inches) Reynolds Wrap® Heavy Duty
   Aluminum Foil
2 small zucchini, sliced
1 medium onion, sliced
1 large tomato, cut in chunks
1 tablespoon olive oil or vegetable oil
3/4 teaspoon lemon pepper seasoning
1/2 teaspoon dried oregano
1/2 teaspoon salt

☆ Preheat oven to 450 degrees or grill to medium-high.
☆ Center vegetables on sheet of Reynolds Wrap®
    Heavy Duty Aluminum Foil.
☆ Drizzle with oil. Sprinkle with seasonings.
☆ Bring up foil sides. Double-fold top and ends to
    seal, making 1 large packet, leaving room for heat
    circulation inside.
☆ Bake 20 to 25 minutes on a cookie sheet in oven, or
    grill 12 to 14 minutes in covered grill.

Serves 4 to 6. Per serving: 51 calories; 3g total fat; 7g carbohydrate; 1g protein; 0mg cholesterol; 244mg sodium

Apples and Rice

1 cup New York State Empire apples, cubed and peeled
1 1/4 cups uncooked brown rice
4 tablespoons butter
2 1/2 cups chunky apple sauce
1/4 cup packed brown sugar
1 3/4 tablespoons ground cinnamon
Dash of salt

☆ Cook rice according to package directions. Stir 2 tablespoons butter in hot rice.
☆ Add applesauce, apples, brown sugar, 1 1/2 tablespoons cinnamon, and salt.
☆ Spoon into greased, deep, 2-quart baking dish.
☆ Dot with remaining butter; sprinkle with remaining cinnamon. Bake uncovered at 350 degrees for 35 minutes or until heated through.

Serves 6 to 8. Per serving: 342 calories; 9.1g total fat; 64.5g carbohydrate; 3.3g protein; 20.7g cholesterol; 4g dietary fiber; 35.75mg sodium

Reprinted with permission from the New York Apple Association.

Bountiful Black Bean Bulgur

1 cup dry bulgur wheat
2 1/2 cups chicken broth or water
1 12-ounce can chickpeas, drained
1 12-ounce can black beans, drained
1/4 cup chopped green onions, sautéed
1 cup chopped red pepper
1 cup chopped, peeled, and seeded cucumber
1 teaspoon Tabasco sauce
1 teaspoon cumin
2 tablespoons chopped fresh cilantro
Salt to taste (if using water)
Optional: 1 can cooked corn, drained

☆ Soak bulgur in chicken broth or water overnight. Drain off any excess liquid.
☆ Sauté onions in a small amount of vegetable oil.
☆ Combine all ingredients in large stir-fry pan and cook until just hot.
☆ Garnish with fresh cilantro.

Serves 6 (main dish) or 10 (side dish). Per serving (side dish): 140 calories; 1g total fat; 27g carbohydrate; 7g protein; 230mg sodium

Brown Rice Medley

2 1/4 cups chicken broth
2 cloves garlic, minced
3 medium carrots, cut diagonally 1/4
1/4 teaspoon fresh ground pepper
1 cup UNCLE BEN'S® Brown Rice — Original Brown
1 cup mushrooms, thinly sliced
1/2 cup green onions, chopped

☆ Combine chicken broth, garlic, carrots, and ground pepper in a medium saucepan.
☆ Bring mixture to boil over medium heat. Add rice.
☆ Cover and simmer over low heat for 25 minutes. Add mushrooms and green onions.
☆ Cover and continue cooking until all liquid is absorbed, about 5 more minutes.

Serves 6. Per serving: 143 calories; 1.4g total fat; 29.2g carbohydrate; 3.8g protein; 0g cholesterol; 2.4g dietary fiber; 570.27mg sodium

Reprinted with permission from Uncle Ben's®.

Lentils and Rice Pilaf

1 tablespoon extra virgin olive oil
2 large onions, peeled and sliced (4 cups)
4 cups low-sodium chicken or vegetable broth
1 cup lentils, dry, washed (2 cups cooked)
1/2 cup long-grain white rice
1/4 teaspoon salt
1/4 teaspoon pepper
2 tablespoons chopped cilantro

☆ Heat the broth in a saucepan. Add the lentils and simmer 20 minutes.
☆ While the lentils are cooking, heat the oil in a large high-sided skillet on medium-high.
☆ Sauté the onions until golden brown.
☆ Take 1/2 the onions out of the pan and set aside.
☆ Add the remaining onions, rice, salt, and pepper to the simmering lentils.
☆ Cover and bring to a boil. Reduce the heat and cook very slowly about 20 minutes or until the lentils and rice are tender.
☆ Serve in a bowl; top with the reserved onions and chopped cilantro.

Serves 4. Per serving: 286 calories; 4g total fat; 49g carbohydrate; 10g dietary fiber; 208mg sodium

Peach Brown Rice

1 can peach halves (15 1/2 ounces) in juice
1 cup UNCLE BEN'S® Brown Rice — Original Brown
1/2 teaspoon ginger, grated, fresh
1/2 teaspoon salt
3/4 cup cashews, chopped

☆ Drain peaches, reserving the juice. Add water to juice
   to make 2 1/4 cups of liquid.
☆ Use this liquid to cook rice according to package
   directions. Simmer 25 minutes.
☆ While rice is simmering, chop enough peaches to
   make 1/2 cup.
☆ Add chopped peaches and ginger to rice. Simmer an
   additional 5 minutes or until liquid is absorbed.
☆ Remove rice to serving dish. Sprinkle with cashews.
   Garnish with reserved peach halves.

Serves 4. Per serving: 373 calories; 13.2g total fat; 58.6g
carbohydrate; 8.3g protein; 0g cholesterol; 4g dietary
fiber; 301.57mg sodium

Reprinted with permission from Uncle Ben's®.

Recipes:
guilt-free extras

Berry Power Drink

1 cup fruit juice (such as orange, cranberry, or apple)

1 cup fresh or frozen strawberries

1 8-ounce carton vanilla low-fat yogurt

2/3 cup Quaker® Oats (quick or old-fashioned variety, uncooked)

1 cup ice cubes

Sugar to taste

☆ Place all ingredients except ice in blender container.

☆ Cover. Blend on high speed about 2 minutes or until smooth.

☆ Gradually add ice; blend on high speed an additional minute or until smooth. Serve immediately.

Serves 1. Per serving (with orange juice): 250 calories; 4.5g total fat; 44g carbohydrate; 11g protein; 5mg cholesterol; 5g dietary fiber; 80mg sodium

Reprinted with permission from The Quaker Oats Company.

Cantaloupe Crush

1/2 cantaloupe

1 cup fat-free milk

1 1/2 cups ice

Sweetener as needed: about 1 to 2 teaspoons of
   sugar or the equivalent in artificial sweetener

☆ Cut cantaloupe into small cubes.

☆ Blend all ingredients until smooth.

☆ Sweeten to taste.

Serves 4. Per serving: 90 calories; 0g total fat; 2mg cholesterol; 1g dietary fiber; 74mg sodium

Frozen Blue Devil

6 ounces pitted dried plums (about 1 cup)
6 tablespoons hot water
32 ounces white grape juice
1 package (10 ounces) frozen sweetened raspberries,
  partially thawed
2 tablespoons fresh lemon juice

☆ In a blender, combine the dried plums and water;
   process until the plums are finely chopped.

☆ Add the grape juice, raspberries, and lemon juice and
   purée until smooth.

☆ Pour into a shallow metal baking pan.

☆ Freeze for 2 hours, stirring every 30 minutes. Freeze
   for about 2 hours longer or until completely frozen.

☆ To serve, let the icee stand at room temperature for
   about 15 minutes or until slightly softened.

☆ Use a metal spoon to scrape across its surface, trans-
   ferring the ice shards to chilled dessert dishes or wine
   glasses without packing them.

Serves 6. Per serving: 225 calories; 0.4g total fat; 57.1g
carbohydrate; 1.4g protein; 0mg cholesterol; 6.4g dietary
fiber; 11mg sodium

Reprinted with permission from the California Dried Plum Board.

Watermelon Smoothie

2 cups seeded watermelon chunks
1 cup cracked ice
1/2 cup plain yogurt
1 to 2 tablespoons sugar
1/2 teaspoon ground ginger
1/8 teaspoon almond extract

☆ Combine all ingredients in blender container.
☆ Blend until smooth.

Serves 2 to 3. Per serving: 113 calories; 1.6g total fat;
21.8g carbohydrate; 4.2g protein; 0.8g dietary fiber;
56.49mg sodium

Lemon Blueberry Oatmeal Muffins

1 3/4 cups Quaker® Oats (quick or old-fashioned, uncooked), divided

2 tablespoons firmly packed brown sugar

1 cup all-purpose flour (add an additional 2 tablespoons if using old-fashioned oats)

1/2 cup granulated sugar

1 tablespoon baking powder

1/4 teaspoon salt (optional)

1 cup skim milk

2 egg whites, lightly beaten

2 tablespoons vegetable oil

1 teaspoon grated lemon peel

1 teaspoon vanilla

1 cup fresh or frozen blueberries (do not thaw)

☆ Heat oven to 400 degrees. Line 12 medium muffin cups with paper baking cups.

☆ For topping, combine 1/4 cup oats and brown sugar; set aside. For muffins, combine 1 1/2 cups oats with remaining dry ingredients in large bowl; mix well.

☆ In small bowl, combine milk, egg whites, oil, lemon peel, and vanilla; mix well. Add to dry ingredients; stir until moistened. Gently stir in berries.

☆ Fill muffin cups almost full; sprinkle with topping.

☆ Bake 20 to 24 minutes or until light golden brown.

☆ Cool muffins in pan on wire rack for five minutes; remove from pan. Serve warm.

Serves 12. Per serving: 168 calories; 3.9g total fat; 29.1g carbohydrate; 5.2g protein; 2.8g dietary fiber; 71.42mg sodium

Reprinted with permission from The Quaker Oats Company.

Low-Fat Pumpkin Bread

Nonstick cooking spray
1 cup Dried Plum Purée*
1 cup packed brown sugar
1 cup granulated sugar
4 large eggs
1 cup (1/2 of 1 16-ounce can) canned pumpkin
2 2/3 cups all-purpose flour
2 teaspoons baking powder
1 teaspoon each baking soda and cinnamon
1/2 teaspoon each salt and ground cloves
1/4 teaspoon each ground ginger and nutmeg

☆ Heat oven to 350 degrees.

☆ Lightly coat two 8 1/2x4 1/2-inch loaf pans with cooking spray; set aside.

☆ In large bowl, blend Dried Plum Purée* with sugars. Beat in eggs and pumpkin just to blend.

☆ In medium bowl, combine flour, baking powder, baking soda, cinnamon, salt, cloves, ginger, and nutmeg.

☆ Add to dried plum mixture, mixing just until moistened.

☆ Spread batter in pans, dividing equally.

☆ Bake in center of oven about 1 hour or until wooden pick inserted in center comes out clean.

☆ Cool in the pan for 10 minutes. Turn onto rack to cool completely.

☆ Breads can be wrapped tightly in foil and frozen up to 1 month.

(continued on next page)

(continued)

*Dried Plum Purée:

☆ In the food processor container, combine 2/3 cup
  (4 ounces) pitted dried plums and 3 tablespoons
  water. Process on and off until finely chopped.
  (Makes 1/2 cup.)

Serves 32. Per serving: 118 calories; 1g total fat; 26g carbohydrate; 2g protein; 27mg cholesterol; 1g dietary fiber;
113mg sodium

Apple "Pan" Cake

1/2 cup cake flour

3 tablespoons sugar

1/2 teaspoon baking soda

1/4 teaspoon ground cinnamon

1/4 teaspoon ground allspice

1 egg, lightly beaten

1/4 cup nonfat or low-fat milk

1 teaspoon salad oil

1 teaspoon lemon juice

1 cup peeled, shredded apple

Pan spray

1/4 cup low-fat sour cream

2 tablespoons brown sugar

☆ In a medium bowl, combine cake flour, sugar, baking soda, and spices and stir until blended.

☆ Beat egg with milk and oil. Sprinkle lemon juice over shredded apple. Combine egg mixture with shredded apple and mix.

☆ Stir apple and flour mixture until just blended.

☆ Heat a 10-inch nonstick sauté pan over medium heat. Spray and add apple batter.

☆ Cook over low to medium heat until just brown on the bottom and sides begin to firm, 5 to 7 minutes.

☆ Flip "pan" cake and cook over low to medium heat until browned and springs back in center with finger touch, about 5 minutes.

(continued on next page)

(continued)

☆ Remove from heat and slide onto serving dish.

☆ Dollop with sour cream, sprinkle with brown sugar, and cut into wedges. Serve while warm.

☆ Optional toppings include maple syrup, honey, fruit jams, cinnamon-sugar, and/or ice cream for a true a la mode apple dessert.

☆ Optional additions to batter include 1/4 cup of chopped walnuts, pecans, almonds, raisins, or other dried fruit.

Serves 6. Per serving: 120 calories; 4g total fat; 19g carbohydrate; 2g protein

Yogurt-Bran Muffins

1/2 cup bran cereal
1/2 cup hot water
2/3 cup packed brown sugar
1/4 cup applesauce
1 egg, slightly beaten
1 cup low-fat vanilla yogurt
1 cup bran cereal
1 cup whole-wheat flour
1 cup cake flour
1 1/4 teaspoons baking soda
1/2 teaspoon salt
1 teaspoon baking powder
Nonstick cooking spray

☆ Preheat oven to 400 degrees. In a small bowl, pour hot water over the bran cereal. Set aside and let stand.

☆ In a large bowl, combine sugar, applesauce, beaten egg, low-fat yogurt, and bran cereal; mix well.

☆ Sift whole-wheat flour, cake flour, soda, baking powder, and salt together and mix with the above ingredients.

☆ Mix the hot water and bran cereal combination into other ingredients; mix until just combined.

☆ Spray a muffin pan with nonstick cooking spray and fill with 1/4 cup batter. Bake for 8 to 10 minutes.

Serves 12. Per serving: 110 calories; 4g total fat; 25g carbohydrate; 4g protein; 330mg sodium

Apple Oat Pancakes

1 medium to large New York State Empire apple,
    cored, peeled, and grated
1 cup quick oats
1 cup skim milk
1 cup plain yogurt
3 eggs
3/4 cup whole-wheat flour
3/4 cup all-purpose flour
3/4 teaspoon baking soda
3/4 teaspoon baking powder
1/4 cup vegetable oil
Pancake syrup

☆ In a large mixing bowl, combine Empire apple, quick
    oats, skim milk, and plain yogurt; stir.
☆ Let sit for 15 minutes. Add eggs and stir to combine.
☆ In another bowl, sift together whole-wheat flour, all-
    purpose flour, baking soda, and baking powder.
☆ Add flour mixture to the apple-oat mixture and stir well.
    Add oil and mix.
☆ Drop by large spoonfuls onto a hot, lightly oiled grid-
    dle; cook over medium heat until well-browned on
    both sides.
☆ Serve with pancake syrup.

Serves 10 to 12. Per serving (1 pancake): 231 calories;
8.6g total fat; 30.7g carbohydrate; 8.6g protein; 3.3g
dietary fiber; 143.79mg sodium

Reprinted with permission from the New York Apple Association.

Cinnamon-Orange Pancakes

3/4 cup all-purpose flour

2 tablespoons wheat germ

1 cup whole-wheat flour

2 teaspoons baking powder

1 tablespoon sugar

1 teaspoon ground cinnamon

1 cup skim milk

3/4 cup fresh orange juice

Egg substitute equivalent to 1 egg

1 teaspoon grated fresh orange peel

Vegetable oil spray

☆ In a medium mixing bowl, combine all dry ingredients and mix until well-blended.

☆ In another medium bowl, combine all liquid ingredients and orange peel. Stir to mix well.

☆ Pour liquid ingredients mixture into dry ingredients and stir only until moistened.

☆ Preheat griddle or skillet for pancakes. Spray lightly with vegetable oil spray.

☆ For each pancake, pour 1/4 cup of batter onto griddle or skillet. Turn each pancake when edges are dry and bubbles appear on top. Serve hot.

Serves 6. Per serving (2 pancakes): 171 calories; 1g total fat; 34g carbohydrate; 7g protein; 1mg cholesterol; 140mg sodium

Reproduced with permission

Recipes

© 2003, Copyright American Heart Association

Barley Pumpkin Waffles

1/2 cup warm water (105 to 115 degrees)
1 package (1/4 ounce) active dry yeast
3 tablespoons granulated sugar, divided
1 3/4 cups all-purpose wheat flour
1/2 cup barley flour
2 tablespoons pumpkin pie spice
1 tablespoon baking soda
1 teaspoon salt
2 cups low-fat buttermilk
1/2 cup prepared solid pack pumpkin
2 tablespoons butter, melted

- ☆ Combine water and 1 teaspoon sugar in small bowl.
- ☆ Sprinkle yeast over water; let stand 5 minutes or until surface bubbles to show yeast is working.
- ☆ Combine flours, remaining sugar, pumpkin pie spice, baking soda, and salt in large bowl; set aside.
- ☆ In small bowl, combine buttermilk, pumpkin, and melted butter.
- ☆ Stir liquid ingredients and yeast mixture into dry ingredients until well-blended.
- ☆ Cover batter and refrigerate overnight.
- ☆ To prepare waffles, heat waffle iron. Pour in 1/2 to 1 cup batter, according to the size of the waffle iron. Bake until waffles are done.

Serves 4. Per serving: 425 calories; 8g total fat; 76g carbohydrate; 13g protein; 20mg cholesterol; 5g dietary fiber; 1718mg sodium

Maple Apple Oatmeal

3 cups apple juice

1/2 teaspoon ground cinnamon

1/4 teaspoon salt (optional)

1 1/2 cups Quaker® Oats (quick or old-fashioned variety, uncooked)

1/2 cup chopped fresh or dried apple

1/4 cup Aunt Jemima® Syrup

1/2 cup chopped nuts (optional)

☆ In medium saucepan, bring juice, cinnamon, and salt to a boil; stir in oats, apple, and syrup.

☆ Return to a boil; reduce heat to medium.

☆ Cook 1 minute for quick oats or 5 minutes for old-fashioned oats or until most of juice is absorbed, stirring occasionally. Stir in nuts, if desired.

☆ Let stand until desired consistency.

Microwave directions:

☆ In 3-quart microwaveable bowl, combine all ingredients except nuts.

☆ Microwave on high 6 to 7 minutes for quick oats and 9 to 10 minutes for old-fashioned oats or until most of juice is absorbed. Stir in nuts, if desired.

☆ Let stand until of desired consistency.

Serves 6. Per serving: 320 calories; 9.4g total fat; 53.35g carbohydrate; 8.22g protein; 0g cholesterol; 5.32g dietary fiber; 112.51mg sodium; 0.27g sugars

Reprinted with permission from The Quaker Oats Company.

Old-Fashioned Barley Pudding

2/3 cup pearl barley

3 cups boiling water

1 teaspoon salt

1 1/3 cups milk

1/8 teaspoon salt

1/4 cup brown sugar

1 tablespoon butter or margarine

1 teaspoon vanilla

2 eggs, lightly beaten

1/2 teaspoon grated lemon rind

1 teaspoon lemon juice

1/3 cup raisins

☆ Boil water and add barley and salt. Cook slowly for 45 minutes or until barley is tender. Cool.

☆ Combine milk, salt, sugar, butter, vanilla, and eggs and beat well. Then add cooked barley, raisins, lemon rind, and juice.

☆ Turn into a well-greased 1 1/2-quart baking pan. Set pan into a larger baking pan in oven.

☆ Pour hot water into the larger pan to within an inch of the top of the custard.

☆ Bake at 325 degrees for about 1 hour until a knife inserted in the center comes out clean.

☆ Serve hot or cold.

Serves 6. Per serving: 201 calories; 4.3g total fat; 35.6g carbohydrate; 6.1g protein; 3.8g dietary fiber; 443.82mg sodium; 0g sugars

Reprinted with permission from the Alberta Barley Commission.

Chickpea Dip with Vegetables

1 12 1/2-ounce can chickpeas, drained, rinsed well

1 cup plain low-fat yogurt (equivalent to 1 8-ounce container of yogurt)

2 tablespoons fresh lemon juice

1/2 tablespoon olive oil

3 drops hot pepper sauce

1 carrot, grated

2 cucumbers, peeled, seeded, and diced

2 Roma tomatoes, finely chopped

1/4 red onion, diced

☆ Blend chickpeas, yogurt, lemon juice, olive oil, and hot sauce in a blender until smooth.

☆ Transfer dip to a shallow serving bowl and pile the colorful vegetables on top, leaving an outer rim of dip to be seen.

☆ Serve with pita bread or toasted wheat bread triangles.

Serves 6. Per serving: 157 calories; 4g total fat; 2mg cholesterol; 5g dietary fiber; 42mg sodium

Onion Dip

1 cup low-fat cottage cheese
1/4 cup finely chopped scallions
2 teaspoons lemon juice

☆ Combine cottage cheese and lemon juice and blend
in the blender.
☆ Add scallions and stir.
☆ For dipping, provide each person with 1/2 cup of
blanched vegetables.

Serves 4. Per serving: 44 calories; 0.6g total fat; 2.2g carbohydrate; 7.1g protein; 0.2g dietary fiber; 230.42mg
sodium; 0g sugars

Zesty Red Bean Dip and Vegetables

1 15-ounce can dark red kidney beans, undrained
1/4 teaspoon garlic salt
1/4 teaspoon black pepper
1/4 teaspoon cumin
1/4 cup fresh dill, roughly chopped
Dash hot sauce
1/4 cup plain low-fat yogurt
1 green bell pepper, hollowed out (with top and
    seeds removed)
1 medium bell pepper, seeded and sliced into strips
1/2 cup grape tomatoes
1/2 cup mini carrots
1/2 cup bite-sized broccoli florets

☆ Discard two tablespoons of liquid from the can of
   beans. Purée remaining liquid and beans, salt, pepper,
   cumin, and hot sauce in a blender.

☆ Stir in yogurt and empty the purée into hollowed-out
   bell pepper.

☆ Set pepper in the center of a medium plate or shallow
   bowl and surround with bell pepper, grape tomatoes,
   carrots, and broccoli florets. Serve.

Serves 4. Per serving: 134 calories; 0.8g total fat; 24g
carbohydrate; 8g protein; 0.9mg cholesterol; 7g dietary
fiber; 455mg sodium

Caribbean Salsa

2 cups chopped seeded watermelon
1 cup chopped fresh pineapple
1 cup chopped onion
1/4 cup chopped fresh cilantro
1/4 cup orange juice
1 tablespoon chopped jalapeño pepper (or to taste)
    or jerk seasoning

☆ In a large bowl, combine ingredients; mix well.
☆ Refrigerate covered at least 1 hour to blend flavors.
☆ Stir before serving.

Serves 8. Per serving: 34 calories; 0g total fat; 1g protein;
0mg cholesterol; 3mg sodium

Fresh Strawberry Relish

2 tablespoons balsamic vinegar

2 tablespoons orange juice

1 tablespoon Dijon-style mustard

1 tablespoon honey

1/2 teaspoon grated orange peel

1/2 teaspoon red pepper flakes

1 pint basket California strawberries, stemmed
    and sliced

3 tablespoons raisins

3 tablespoons chopped walnuts

☆ In medium bowl, measure all ingredients except strawberries, raisins, and walnuts.

☆ Whisk to blend thoroughly.

☆ Add remaining ingredients; toss.

☆ Serve with baked or grilled fish or chicken.

Serves 4. Per serving: 104 calories; 4g total fat; 17g carbohydrate; 2.2g protein; 0mg cholesterol; 114mg sodium.

Watermelon Raspberry Vinaigrette

1 cup cubed seeded watermelon
1/2 cup fresh or frozen raspberries
2 tablespoons honey
1 tablespoon raspberry vinegar

☆ In blender or food processor, process watermelon and raspberries until liquefied.

☆ Add honey and vinegar; pulse until blended.

☆ Cover and store in refrigerator.

☆ Shake well before using.

Serves 8. Per serving (2 tablespoons): 27 calories; 0.1g total fat; 7g carbohydrate; 0.21g protein; 0mg cholesterol; 1g dietary fiber; 1mg sodium

Honey Berry Butter

1 pint California strawberries, washed and stemmed
1 tablespoon lemon juice
1/2 cup orange honey

☆ In blender, whirl berries until smooth.
☆ Measure 2 cups purée into saucepan. Add remaining ingredients.
☆ Bring to boil, then simmer 20 to 30 minutes, stirring occasionally. Cool. (This is a butter that will pour.)

Per recipe (1 1/2 cups): 100 calories; 0g total fat; 30g carbohydrate; 0g protein; 0mg cholesterol; 1g dietary fiber; 2mg sodium

20-20-20 food lists: calorie counting at a glance

Look through this extensive list of foods, where the calories are figured for you. Use it to make substitutions in your own meal plan and to add variety to your daily diet.

This list sorts items by calories within each food group, but don't count on calories alone to make your choices. Be sure you consider the nutritional value of foods you choose. Watching calories may help you lose weight, but eating a nutritious diet is essential to your overall health.

Here are a few more points to help you use this list more effectively.

■ Meat weights, unless otherwise noted, refer to servings that are cooked, not raw.

■ Calorie counts for items given as "from recipe" are based on typical ingredients. They won't, however, be accurate for every possible recipe for a given dish.

■ Foods listed as "commercial" are already prepared items you can buy from your local store. "Fast food" items, of course, come from fast food restaurants.

■ Unless otherwise noted, individual fruits and vegetables are of medium size.

■ When the amount is given as "1 serving," check the package or the recipe to determine what that means.

■ Oils are not included in this list, as they all have about the same count of 120 calories per tablespoon.

With this food list and the information you've gained throughout this book, you're ready to take charge of your fitness.

20 Grains
under 50 calories

Coffee substitute prepared with water	8 ounces	12
Toasted wheat germ	1 tbl	27
Air-popped popcorn	1 cup	31
Cheese crackers with peanut butter	1 sandwich	34
Brown rice snack cake	1 cake	35
Wheat crackers with peanut butter	1 sandwich	35
Rye wafers	1 wafer	37
Popcorn snack cake	1 cake	38
Wheat crackers	4 crackers	38
Saltine crackers	3 crackers	39
Cheese crackers	8 1"-square crackers	40
Puffed wheat cereal	1 cup	44
Animal crackers	4 crackers	44
Cooked oat bran	1/2 cup	44
Low-calorie wheat bread	1 slice	46
Low-calorie oat bran bread	1 slice	46
Low-calorie rye bread	1 slice	47
Seasoned croutons	1/4 cup	47
Low-calorie white bread	1 slice	48
Oyster crackers	1/4 cup	49

20 Grains
50 - 100 calories

Buttermilk biscuit, from recipe	1-1/2" biscuit	50
Italian bread	1 slice	54
Oil-popped popcorn	1 cup	55
Puffed rice cereal	1 cup	56
Corn tortilla	1 tortilla	58
Graham crackers	2 squares	59
Baked taco shell	1 shell	62
White bread	1 slice	67
Sourdough bread	1/2" slice	68
Whole-wheat bread	1 slice	69
Raisin bread	1 slice	71
Whole-wheat crackers	4 crackers	71
Pancake from mix	1 pancake	74
White pita	4" pita	77
Plain melba toast	4 crackers	78
Plain frozen pancake	1 pancake	82
Rye bread	1 slice	83
Low-fat frozen waffle	1 waffle	83
Plain frozen waffle	1 waffle	87
Instant corn grits	1 packet	89

20 Grains
100 - 150 calories

Corn flakes	1 cup	101
Plain instant Cream of Wheat	1 packet	102
Plain instant oatmeal	1 packet	104
Kellogg's Product 19 cereal	1 cup	109
General Mills Cheerios cereal	1 cup	111
Kellogg's Frosted Flakes cereal	1 cup	114
Egg bread	1 slice	115
Kellogg's Special K cereal	1 cup	117
Malt-O-Meal cooked with water	1 cup	122
Hamburger or hotdog roll	1 roll	123
Instant apple cinnamon oatmeal	1 packet	125
Frozen French toast	1 slice	126
Quick Cream of Wheat cooked with water	1 cup	129
Regular Cream of Wheat cooked with water	1 cup	133
Plain English muffin	1 muffin	134
Plain hard granola bar	1 bar	134
Plain tortilla chips	1 ounce	142
Quick-cooking corn grits	1 cup	145
Oatmeal cooked with water	1 cup	145
Commercial flour tortilla	8" tortilla	146

20 Grains
150 - 200 calories

Cooked bulgur	1 cup	151
Instant maple oatmeal	1 packet	153
Shredded wheat cereal	2 biscuits	156
Kellogg's All-Bran cereal	1 cup	156
Instant white long-grain rice	1 cup	162
White pita	6-1/2" pita	165
Raisin bran cereal	1 cup	171
Cooked whole-wheat spaghetti	1 cup	174
Cooked couscous	1 cup	176
Bread stuffing, from mix	1/2 cup	178
Corn muffin, from recipe	1 muffin	180
Commercial blueberry muffin	1 small muffin	183
Kellogg's Low-fat Granola	1/2 cup	186
Frosted, bite-size, mini-wheat cereal	1 cup	189
Cinnamon raisin bagel	3" bagel	189
Plain bagel	3" bagel	190
Egg bagel	3" bagel	192
Cooked pearl barley	1 cup	193
Banana bread, from recipe	1 slice	196
Cooked spaghetti or macaroni	1 cup	197

20 Grains
over 200 calories

Kellogg's Strawberry Pop Tart	1 pastry	205
Regular white long-grain rice, cooked	1 cup	205
Lender's Premium Blueberry Bagel	3" bagel	209
Spinach egg noodles, cooked	1 cup	211
Buttermilk biscuit, from recipe	2-1/2" biscuit	212
Eggo Banana Bread Waffle	1 serving	212
Egg noodles, cooked	1 cup	213
Brown long-grain rice, cooked	1 cup	216
Plain waffle, from recipe	1 waffle	218
Baked puff pastry, from frozen	1 shell	223
Hard salted pretzels	10 pretzels	229
Croissant	1 croissant	231
Chinese chow mein noodles	1 cup	237
Regular white short-grain rice, cooked	1 cup	242
Fast food hush puppies	5 pieces	257
Kraft Macaroni and Cheese, from mix	1 cup	259
Cinnamon raisin bagel	4-1/2" bagel	359
Plain bagel	4-1/2" bagel	360
Egg bagel	4-1/2" bagel	364
Fast food pancakes with butter and syrup	2 pancakes	520

20 Fruits
under 50 calories

Fresh strawberries	1 berry	4
Sun-dried tomato	1 piece	5
Fresh apricot	1 apricot	17
Fresh cantaloupe	1/8 melon	24
Ripe canned olives	5 olives	25
Fresh tomato	1 tomato	26
Canned pineapple in juice	1 slice	28
Red or green grapes	10 grapes	36
Fresh plum	1 plum	36
Pink or red grapefruit	1/2 grapefruit	37
Tangerine	1 tangerine	37
Canned pears in juice	1/2 pear	38
Canned pineapple in syrup	1 slice	38
Canned tomato juice	1 cup	41
Fresh peach	1 peach	42
Canned peaches in juice	1/2 peach	43
Canned whole tomatoes	1 cup	46
Fresh kiwi	1 kiwi fruit	46
Watermelon	1 cup	49
Fresh cherries	10 cherries	49

20 Fruits
50 - 100 calories

Fresh strawberries	1 cup	50
California avocado	1 ounce	50
Honeydew	1/8 melon	56
Canned pears in syrup	1/2 pear	56
Fresh raspberries	1 cup	60
Orange	1 orange	62
Nectarine	1 nectarine	67
Canned stewed tomatoes	1 cup	71
Canned peaches in syrup	1/2 peach	73
Canned tomato sauce	1 cup	74
Fresh blackberries	1 cup	75
Fresh pineapple	1 cup	76
Dried apples	5 rings	78
Fresh blueberries	1 cup	81
Fresh apple with skin	1 apple	81
Dried apricots	10 halves	84
Canned cranberry sauce	2-ounce slice	86
Canned unsweetened grapefruit juice	1 cup	94
Dried figs	2 figs	97
Fresh pear	1 pear	98

20 Fruits
100 - 150 calories

Dried prunes	5 prunes	100
Canned unsweetened orange juice	1 cup	105
Canned unsweetened applesauce	1 cup	105
Fresh banana	1 banana	109
Canned fruit cocktail in juice	1 cup	109
Canned peaches in juice	1 cup	109
Raisins	1/4 cup	109
Orange juice, fresh or from frozen concentrate	1 cup	112
Fresh grapes	1 cup	114
Dates	5 dates	114
Canned sweetened grapefruit juice	1 cup	115
Canned or bottled unsweetened apple juice	1 cup	117
Canned apricots in juice	1 cup	117
Fresh papaya	1 papaya	119
Canned pears in juice	1 cup	124
Canned pineapple-orange drink	8 fluid ounces	125
Sweetened grape juice, from frozen concentrate	1 cup	128
Fresh mango	1 mango	135
Bottled cranberry juice cocktail	8 fluid ounces	144
Canned pineapple in juice	1 cup	149

20 Fruits
over 150 calories

Canned grapefruit sections in syrup	1 cup	152
Canned tangerines in syrup	1 cup	154
Canned or bottled unsweetened grape juice	1 cup	154
Avocado	1/2 avocado	162
Canned fruit cocktail in heavy syrup	1 cup	181
Canned prune juice	1 cup	182
Frozen sweetened blueberries	1 cup	186
Canned sweetened applesauce	1 cup	194
Canned peaches in heavy syrup	1 cup	194
Canned pears in heavy syrup	1 cup	197
Canned pineapple in heavy syrup	1 cup	199
Canned apricots in heavy syrup	1 cup	214
Canned tomato paste	1 cup	215
Raw plantain	1 plantain	218
Frozen sweetened peaches	1 cup	235
Frozen sweetened strawberries	1 cup	245
Frozen sweetened mixed fruit	1 cup	245
Frozen sweetened raspberries	1 cup	258
Stewed prunes without sugar	1 cup	265
Frozen cooked rhubarb with sugar	1 cup	278

20 Vegetables
under 15 calories

Radish	1 radish	1
Raw green pepper	1 ring	3
Raw cauliflower	1 floweret	3
Raw garlic	1 clove	4
Raw green or spring onions	1 whole onion	5
Raw onion	1 medium slice	5
Raw celery	1 stalk	6
Raw spinach	1 cup	7
Iceberg lettuce	1 cup	7
Canned beets	1 beet	7
Romaine lettuce	1 cup	8
Raw endive	1 cup	9
Raw broccoli	1 spear	9
Canned hearts of palm	1 piece	9
Raw alfalfa sprouts	1 cup	10
Boiled broccoli	1 spear	10
Dried shiitake mushrooms	1 mushroom	11
Dill pickle	1 pickle	12
Cucumber	1 cup	14
Canned or fresh boiled asparagus	4 spears	14

20 Vegetables
15 - 40 calories

Raw button mushrooms	1 cup	18
Raw cabbage	1 cup	18
Boiled mustard greens	1 cup	21
Raw summer squash	1 cup	23
Peeled cucumber	1 cucumber	24
Raw broccoli	1 cup	25
Raw cauliflower	1 cup	25
Canned green beans	1 cup	27
Boiled eggplant	1 cup	28
Boiled cauliflower	1 cup	29
Boiled turnip greens	1 cup	29
Raw carrot	1 carrot	31
Raw green or red pepper	1 pepper	32
Boiled turnips	1 cup	33
Boiled cabbage	1 cup	33
Boiled summer squash	1 cup	36
Boiled kale	1 cup	36
Canned carrots	1 cup	37
Canned mushrooms	1 cup	37
Boiled green beans, from frozen	1 cup	38

20 Vegetables
40 - 60 calories

Chopped raw green or red pepper	1 cup	40
Boiled spinach	1 cup	41
Raw onion	1 onion	42
Boiled broccoli	1 cup	44
Boiled green beans	1 cup	44
Canned sauerkraut	1 cup	45
Canned vegetable juice cocktail	1 cup	46
Raw carrots	1 cup	47
Boiled kohlrabi	1 cup	48
Boiled pumpkin	1 cup	49
Boiled turnip or collard greens	1 cup	49
Canned spinach	1 cup	49
Boiled asparagus	1 cup	50
Boiled okra	1 cup	52
Chopped cooked broccoli, from frozen	1 cup	52
Boiled carrots, from frozen	1 cup	53
Canned beets	1 cup	53
Chopped cooked spinach, from frozen	1 cup	53
Boiled mixed vegetables, from frozen	1/2 cup	54
Boiled corn on the cob, from frozen	1 ear	59

20 Vegetables
60 - 100 calories

Boiled artichoke	1 artichoke	60
Raw onion	1 cup	61
Boiled brussels sprouts	1 cup	61
Chopped, boiled collard greens, from frozen	1 cup	61
Hashed brown potatoes, from frozen	1 patty	63
Boiled brussels sprouts, from frozen	1 cup	65
Boiled rutabagas	1 cup	66
Fast food mashed potatoes	1/3 cup	66
Canned Chinese water chestnuts	1 cup	70
Boiled carrots	1 cup	70
Boiled beets	1 cup	75
Canned mixed vegetables	1 cup	77
Baked yam	1/2 cup	79
Cooked shiitake mushrooms	1 cup	80
Baked winter squash	1 cup	80
Mashed potatoes with whole milk	1/2 cup	81
Boiled fresh corn on the cob	1 ear	83
Canned pumpkin	1 cup	83
Boiled winter squash, from frozen	1 cup	94
Canned carrot juice	1 cup	94

20 Vegetables
over 100 calories

Baked sweet potato	1 potato	117
Potatoes au gratin, from mix	1 serving	127
Boiled corn, from frozen	1 cup	131
Boiled potatoes	1 potato	144
Fast food coleslaw	3/4 cup	147
Fast food hashed brown potatoes	1/2 cup	151
Canned succotash	1 cup	161
Baked potato	1 potato	161
Canned corn	1 cup	166
Canned cream-style corn	1 cup	184
Canned sweet potato	1 cup	212
Spinach soufflé, from recipe	1 cup	219
Mashed potatoes with whole milk and margarine	1 cup	223
Mashed potatoes, from flakes, whole milk, butter	1 cup	237
Fried onion rings	8-9 rings	276
Fast food French fries	1 small serving	291
Hashed brown potatoes, from recipe	1 cup	323
Boiled, mashed sweet potato	1 cup	344
Fast food French fries	1 medium serving	458
Fast food French fries	1 large serving	578

20 Dairy
under 100 calories

Whipped cream, pressurized	1 tbl	8
Powdered creamer	1 tsp	11
Dessert topping, frozen	1 tbl	13
Half and half	1 tbl	20
Reduced-fat cultured sour cream	1 tbl	20
Grated parmesan cheese	1 tbl	23
Cultured sour cream	1 tbl	26
Fat-free cream cheese	1 ounce	27
Light whipping cream	1 tbl	44
Low-fat cheddar or Colby cheese	1 ounce	49
Heavy whipping cream	1 tbl	52
Kraft Velveeta Light Cheese	1 ounce	62
Neufchatel cheese	1 ounce	74
Feta cheese	1 ounce	75
Part-skim, low-moisture mozzarella cheese	1 ounce	79
Whole-milk mozzarella cheese	1 ounce	80
Dry, nonfat instant milk	1/3 cup	82
Skim milk	1 cup	86
Light vanilla ice cream	1/2 cup	92
Cream cheese	1 ounce	99

20 Dairy
100 – 150 calories

Provolone cheese	1 ounce	100
Blue cheese	1 ounce	100
Butter	1 tbl	102
Corn oil, margarine/butter blend	1 tbl	102
Low-fat milk (1% milkfat)	1 cup	102
Muenster cheese	1 ounce	104
Swiss cheese	1 ounce	107
Ready-to-serve cheese sauce	1/4 cup	110
Cheddar cheese	1 ounce	114
Soft-serve vanilla frozen yogurt	1/2 cup	114
Soft-serve chocolate frozen yogurt	1/2 cup	115
Reduced-fat milk (2% milkfat)	1 cup	122
Nonfat cottage cheese	1 cup	123
Plain skim-milk yogurt (13 grams protein)	8 ounces	127
Vanilla ice cream	1/2 cup	133
Plain whole-milk yogurt (8 grams protein)	8 ounces	138
Regular vanilla pudding from mix (2% milk)	1/2 cup	141
Chocolate ice cream	1/2 cup	143
Plain low-fat yogurt (12 grams protein)	8 ounces	143
Ready-to-eat vanilla pudding	4 ounces	147

20 Dairy
over 150 calories

Ready-to-eat chocolate pudding	4 ounces	150
Chocolate pudding from mix (2% milk)	1/2 cup	155
Low-fat chocolate milk	1 cup	158
Low-fat cottage cheese (1% milkfat)	1 cup	163
Reduced-fat chocolate milk	1 cup	180
Soft-serve French vanilla ice cream	1/2 cup	185
Canned evaporated nonfat milk	1 cup	200
Low-fat cottage cheese (2% milkfat)	1 cup	203
Chocolate milk	1 cup	208
Cottage cheese	1 cup	216
Chocolate milk, from powder (whole milk)	1 cup	226
Low-fat fruit yogurt (10 grams protein)	8 ounces	232
Fast food hot fudge sundae	1 sundae	284
Canned evaporated milk	1 cup	338
Part-skim ricotta cheese	1 cup	339
Eggnog	1 cup	343
Fast food vanilla shake	16 ounces	370
Fast food chocolate shake	16 ounces	423
Whole-milk ricotta cheese	1 cup	428
Canned sweetened condensed milk	1 cup	982

20 Legumes
under 100 calories

Boiled peas in pod	1/2 cup	34
Firm tofu	1/4 cup	49
Canned green peas	1/2 cup	59
Stir-fried mung bean sprouts	1 cup	62
Boiled green peas, from frozen	1/2 cup	63
Morningstar Farms Black Bean Burgers	1 serving	63
Boiled fresh green peas	1/2 cup	67
Miso	1/2 cup	71
Soft tofu	1/4 cup	76
Soy milk	1 cup	81
Boiled peas in pod, from frozen	1 cup	83
Canned split pea soup	1/2 cup	83
Boiled fordhook lima beans, from frozen	1/2 cup	86
Canned blackeyed peas	1/2 cup	93
Canned crowder peas	1/2 cup	93
Hummus	4 tbl	93
Chunky peanut butter	1 tbl	94
Smooth peanut butter	1 tbl	95
Boiled baby lima beans, from frozen	1/2 cup	95
Canned lima beans	1/2 cup	96

20 Legumes
over 100 calories

Boiled black-eyed peas, from dried	1/2 cup	100
Boiled great northern beans, from dried	1/2 cup	105
Boiled lima beans, from dried	1/2 cup	108
Canned red kidney beans	1/2 cup	109
Boiled black-eyed peas, from frozen	1/2 cup	112
Boiled red kidney beans, from dried	1/2 cup	113
Boiled black beans, from dried	1/2 cup	114
Boiled lentils, from dried	1/2 cup	115
Boiled split peas, from dried	1/2 cup	116
Boiled pinto beans, from dried	1/2 cup	117
Canned baked beans	1/2 cup	118
Canned refried beans	1/2 cup	119
Canned baked beans with pork	1/2 cup	124
Boiled green soybeans	1/2 cup	127
Boiled navy beans, from dried	1/2 cup	129
Canned garbanzo beans	1/2 cup	143
Canned white beans	1/2 cup	154
Dry-roasted peanuts	1 ounce	166
Canned baked beans with franks	1/2 cup	184
Roasted soybeans	1/4 cup	203

20 Fish
under 150 calories

Steamed shrimp	6 large shrimp	33
Fish stock, from recipe	1 cup	40
Grilled or broiled orange roughy	3 ounces	76
Steamed Alaska king crab	3 ounces	82
Steamed lobster	3 ounces	83
Imitation crab meat	3 ounces	87
Grilled or broiled cod	3 ounces	89
Grilled or broiled haddock	3 ounces	95
Canned light tuna in water	3 ounces	99
Grilled or broiled flounder or sole	3 ounces	99
Smoked salmon	3 ounces	100
Grilled or broiled perch	3 ounces	103
Canned white tuna in water	3 ounces	109
Fried shrimp	6 large shrimp	109
Broiled or grilled red snapper	3 ounces	109
Canned salmon	3 ounces	118
Broiled or grilled yellowfin tuna	3 ounces	118
Broiled or grilled halibut	3 ounces	119
Broiled or grilled swordfish	3 ounces	132
Broiled or grilled farm-raised rainbow trout	3 ounces	144

20 Fish
over 150 calories

Canned sardines in tomato sauce	3 ounces	153
Fish sticks, from frozen	2 sticks	155
Poached wild coho salmon	3 ounces	156
Canned clam chowder prepared with milk	1 cup	164
Canned tuna in oil	3 ounces	168
Fried oysters	6 oysters	173
Broiled or grilled Atlantic farmed salmon	3 ounces	175
Canned sardines in oil	3 ounces	177
Broiled or grilled sockeye salmon	3 ounces	184
Kippered herring	3 ounces	185
Blue crab cakes	2 cakes	186
Fried catfish	3 ounces	195
Fried scallops	6 large scallops	200
Fried fish fillet	3 ounces	211
Pickled herring	3 ounces	223
Steamed oysters	6 oysters	246
Tuna salad, from recipe	1 cup	383
Fast food fish sandwich with tartar sauce	1 sandwich	431
Fast food fried clams	3/4 cup	451
Fast food fried shrimp	6-8 shrimp	454

20 Meats
under 100 calories

Beef broth, from one bouillon cube	6 ounces	5
Chicken broth, from one bouillon cube	6 ounces	9
Beef broth, from condensed	1 cup	29
Simmered chicken liver	1 liver	31
Chicken broth, from condensed	1 cup	39
Liquid egg substitute	1/4 cup	53
Turkey bacon	3 slices	53
Poached egg	1 medium	66
Deli fat-free roasted chicken breast	3 ounces	68
Beef or pork salami	1 ounce	71
Poached egg	1 large egg	75
Roasted chicken drumstick, no skin	1 drumstick	76
Hard-boiled egg	1 large egg	78
Stewed chicken meat	3 ounces	79
Poached egg	1 extra-large egg	86
Boiled ham	3 ounces	89
Fried egg	1 large egg	92
Cooked fresh pork sausage	2 links	96
Deli rotisserie turkey breast	3 ounces	96
Roasted chicken wing with skin	1 wing	99

20 Meats
100 - 150 calories

Cooked fresh pork sausage	1-ounce patty	100
Scrambled egg	1 large egg	101
Turkey frankfurter	1 frank	102
Cooked fresh pork and beef sausage	2 links	103
Roasted skinless, boneless chicken thigh	1 thigh	109
Pork bacon	3 medium slices	109
Turkey ham	3 ounces	109
Extra lean ham	3 ounces	111
Chicken frankfurter	1 frank	116
Canned cream of chicken soup with water	1 cup	117
Floured and fried chicken drumstick with skin	1 drumstick	120
Roasted white-meat turkey, no skin	3 ounces	132
Beef and pork frankfurter	1 frank	135
Oscar Mayer pork and turkey Little Smokies	5 links	135
Canned chicken in broth	3 ounces	141
Canned ham	3 ounces	142
Roasted boneless, skinless chicken breast	1/2 breast	142
Roasted beef eye of round, no fat	3 ounces	143
Beef frankfurter	1 frank	147
Roasted Cornish game hen, no skin	1/2 hen	147

20 Meats
150 - 200 calories

Cured beef breakfast strips	3 slices	153
Roasted dark-meat turkey, no skin	3 ounces	157
Battered and fried chicken wings with skin	1 wing	159
Fried skinless chicken breast	3 ounces	161
Broiled t-bone steak, no fat	3 ounces	161
Roasted whole leg of lamb, no fat	3 ounces	162
Floured and fried chicken thigh with skin	1 thigh	162
Broiled beef top sirloin	3 ounces	166
Country-style center-sliced cured ham	3 ounces	166
Broiled loin pork chops	3 ounces	172
Grilled Canadian bacon	3 ounces	172
Pork and beef bologna	2 slices	177
Braised beef bottom round	3 ounces	178
Roasted fresh ham	3 ounces	179
Pan-fried beef liver	3 ounces	184
Roasted center loin rib pork roast	3 ounces	190
Jimmy Dean Frozen Sausage Biscuit	1 sandwich	192
Battered and fried chicken drumstick with skin	1 drumstick	193
Roasted beef ribs	3 ounces	195
Pan-fried center loin pork chops	3 ounces	197

20 Meats
200 - 250 calories

Broiled boneless lamb chops	3 ounces	200
Cooked ground turkey	3 ounces	202
Pan-broiled ground bison	3 ounces	202
Broiled center loin pork chops	3 ounces	204
Roasted whole ham	3 ounces	207
Braised fresh pork shoulder	3 ounces	211
Broiled 85%-lean ground beef patty	3 ounces	213
Canned corned beef	3 ounces	213
Braised beef chuck roast	3 ounces	213
Roasted center rib pork roast	3 ounces	217
Canned beef stew	1 cup	218
Broiled beef top sirloin	3 ounces	219
Battered and fried chicken breast with skin	3 ounces	221
Broiled 80%-lean ground beef patty	3 ounces	230
Braised beef bottom round	3 ounces	234
Pan-fried center loin pork chops	3 ounces	235
Broiled 75%-lean ground beef patty	3 ounces	236
Battered and fried chicken thigh with skin	1 thigh	238
Fast food hot dog	1 sandwich	242
Simmered turkey giblets	1 cup	242

20 Meats
over 250 calories

Canned chili with beans and meat	1 cup	255
Fast food regular hamburger with condiments	1 sandwich	272
Braised pork shoulder	3 ounces	280
Roasted beef tenderloin	3 ounces	282
Braised beef chuck roast	3 ounces	292
Braised lamb shoulder	3 ounces	294
Fast food regular cheeseburger with condiments	1 sandwich	295
Fast food chili dog	1 sandwich	296
Roasted beef ribs	3 ounces	304
Pork braunschweiger	3 ounces	306
Roasted pork back ribs	3 ounces	315
Fast food fried chicken nuggets	6 pieces	319
Braised pork spareribs	3 ounces	337
Fast food roast beef sandwich	1 sandwich	346
Fast food taco	1 small taco	369
Roasted duck	1/2 duck	444
Corndog	1 corndog	460
Chicken pot pie, from frozen	1 small pie	484
Fast food taco	1 large taco	568
Fast food double-patty hamburger with condiments	1 sandwich	576

20 Nuts & Seeds

Dried sesame seeds	1 tbl	47
Dried pine nuts	1 tbl	49
Flaxseed	1 tbl	59
Cashew butter	1 tbl	94
Roasted pumpkin seeds	1 ounce	148
Fresh coconut	1-1/2 ounces	159
Dried pine nuts	1 ounce	160
Dry-roasted pistachios	1 ounce	161
Dry-roasted cashews	1 ounce	163
Almonds	1 ounce	164
Dry-roasted sunflower seeds	1 ounce	165
Honey-roasted almonds	1 ounce	168
Hazelnuts	1 ounce	178
English walnuts	1 ounce	185
Dried Brazil nuts	1 ounce	186
Dry-roasted sunflower seeds	1/4 cup	186
Pecans	1 ounce	196
Dry-roasted macadamia nuts	1 ounce	203
Roasted chestnuts	1 cup	350
Dried sweetened coconut	1 cup	466

20 Sweets & Snacks
under 50 calories

Diet cola	12 fluid ounces	4
Sugar-free gelatin prepared with water	1/2 cup	8
Brown sugar	1 tsp	12
Vanilla extract	1 tsp	12
Cocoa powder	1 tbl	12
Gumdrops	1 piece	16
Granulated sugar	1 tsp	16
Low-fat vanilla wafers	1 cookie	18
Commercial butter cookies	1 cookie	23
Low-calorie pancake syrup	1 tbl	25
Apple butter	1 tbl	29
Powdered sugar	1 tbl	31
Commercial fat-free oatmeal cookies	1 cookie	36
Chocolate-covered raisins	10 pieces	39
Commercial shortbread cookies	1 cookie	40
Ice pops	2-fluid-ounce bar	42
Commercial low-fat chocolate chip cookies	1 cookie	45
Blackstrap molasses	1 tbl	47
Chocolate sandwich cookie with crème filling	1 cookie	47
Sugar-free cocoa mix powder	1/2-ounce envelope	48

20 Sweets & Snacks
50 - 100 calories

Cheese crackers	10 crackers	50
Chocolate syrup	1 tbl	52
Glazed yeast donut holes	1 hole	52
Maple syrup	1 tbl	52
Jam and preserves	1 tbl	56
Fig cookies	1 bar	56
Pancake syrup	1 tbl	57
Cake donut holes	1 hole	59
Honey	1 tbl	64
Oatmeal raisin cookies, from recipe	1 cookie	65
Sugar cookies, from recipe with margarine	1 cookie	66
Chocolate fudge, from recipe	1 piece	70
Commercial peanut butter cookies	1 cookie	72
Commercial sugar cookies	1 cookie	72
Commercial angel food cake	1 piece	72
Chocolate chip cookies, from recipe with margarine	1 cookie	78
Fat-free commercial pound cake	1 slice	79
Gelatin prepared with water	1/2 cup	80
Chocolate nut fudge, from recipe	1 piece	89
Peanut butter cookies, from recipe	1 cookie	95

20 Sweets & Snacks
100 - 200 calories

Jellybeans	10 large pieces	104
Commercial pound cake	1 serving	109
Commercial oatmeal cookie	1 cookie	113
Chocolate chip granola bar	1 bar	119
Low-fat nacho tortilla chips	1 ounce	126
Low-fat potato chips	1 ounce	134
Barbecue potato chips	1 ounce	139
Tortilla chips	1 ounce	142
Lemon-lime soda	12 fluid ounces	147
Sour cream and onion potato chips	1 ounce	151
Cola with caffeine	12 fluid ounces	152
Potato chips	1 ounce	152
Corn chips	1 ounce	153
Pork skins	1 ounce	155
Crème-filled sponge cakes	1 snack cake	155
Cheese puff snacks	1 ounce	157
Grape soda	12 fluid ounces	160
Orange soda	12 fluid ounces	179
Crème-filled chocolate cupcake	1 cupcake	188
Plain cake donut	1 donut	198

20 Sweets & Snacks
200 - 300 calories

Orange sherbet	1 cup	204
Chocolate-covered peanuts	10 pieces	208
German chocolate brownie, from recipe	2" square	221
Commercial cinnamon sweet roll with raisins	1 roll	223
Milk chocolate candy bar	1.55-ounce bar	226
Commercial brownies	1 brownie	227
Commercial pumpkin pie	1 serving	229
Reese's Pieces candy	1/4 cup	234
Commercial chocolate cake with frosting	1 serving	235
Almond Joy candy bar	1 regular bar	235
Glazed yeast donuts	1 donut	242
Fast food brownie	2" square	243
Commercial cheesecake	1 serving	257
Commercial cinnamon coffeecake	1 serving	263
Commercial Danish fruit pastry	1 pastry	263
Gingerbread cake, from recipe	1 serving	263
White cake, from recipe without frosting	1 serving	264
Commercial Danish cheese pastry	1 pastry	266
Commercial coconut custard pie	1 serving	270
Commercial apple pie	1 serving	277

20 Sweets & Snacks
over 300 calories

Commercial lemon meringue pie	1 serving	303
Commercial cherry pie	1 serving	304
Pumpkin pie, from recipe	1 serving	316
Fast food Danish fruit pastry	1 pastry	335
Chocolate cake, from recipe without frosting	1 serving	340
Commercial chocolate crème pie	1 serving	344
Fast food cinnamon Danish pastry	1 pastry	349
Trail mix with chocolate chips, nuts, and seeds	1/2 cup	353
Cherry cheesecake, from recipe	1 serving	356
Blueberry pie, from recipe	1 serving	360
Lemon meringue pie, from recipe	1 serving	362
Pineapple upside-down cake, from recipe	1 serving	367
Commercial fried fruit pies	1 pie	404
Apple pie, from recipe	1 serving	411
Commercial pecan pie	1 serving	452
Cherry pie, from recipe	1 serving	486
Klondike Bar (chocolate-covered vanilla ice cream)	1 bar	488
Pecan pie, from recipe	1 serving	503
Tropical trail mix	1 cup	570
Semisweet chocolate chips	1 cup	805

Recipe index

Index

A

Abdominals
  exercises for 128–129, 211–212
  illustration of 130
Aerobic exercise, *see* Aerobics
Aerobics 159–172
  calories burned during 230
  chest pains and 161
  for atherosclerosis 161–162
  for depression 161
  for diabetes 161
  for fibromyalgia 118
  for high blood pressure 161–162
  for higher metabolism 160
  for weight control 160–161
  See also Water aerobics
Age-related macular degeneration
  (AMD), *see* Macular degeneration
Alcohol
  atherosclerosis and 42, 58
  cancer and 72
  cataracts and 42
  diabetes and 42
  forgetfulness and 42
  weight control and 42
Alzheimer's disease 67–69
Anaerobic exercise 160
  See also Aerobic exercise
Anger management
  for anxiety 106
  for atherosclerosis 106
  for cancer 106
  for depression 106
  for high blood pressure 106
  for stress 106

Angina, *see* Atherosclerosis
Antioxidants
  for Alzheimer's disease 68
  for atherosclerosis 78–80
  for cancer 72–73
  for macular degeneration 81
  for osteoporosis 88
  for rheumatoid arthritis 89
  for skin care 94
  free radicals and 2–3, 19–20, 72–73
Apples
  for atherosclerosis 79
  for weight control 254
Arm muscles, *see* Biceps *and*
  Triceps
Aromatherapy, for depression 110
Arteriosclerosis, *see* Atherosclerosis
Arthritis, *see* Osteoarthritis *and*
  Rheumatoid arthritis
Artificial sweeteners
  arthritis and 42
  migraines and 42
  See also Aspartame *and*
  Saccharin
Asian diet
  beans and 59
  fish and 59
  for atherosclerosis 58–60
  for high cholesterol 58–60
  whole grains and 58
Aspartame
  forgetfulness and 42
  See also Artificial sweeteners
Aspirin, for atherosclerosis 79
Asthma 70–72

Atherosclerosis 77–80
    waist size and 234
Atkins diet, *see* High-protein diets

B

B vitamins
    for Alzheimer's disease 67
    for atherosclerosis 92
    for depression 16
    for insomnia 99
    for osteoarthritis 83
    for stroke 92
    See also Folate, Niacin, Riboflavin, Thiamin, Vitamin B6, *and* Vitamin B12
Bad breath, *see* Gum disease
Ballroom dancing
    calories burned during 230
    classes for 223
    for aerobic exercise 223
    for balance 223
    for flexibility 223
    for muscles 222
    See also Dancing
Beans
    for atherosclerosis 28
    for colon cancer 28
    for constipation 28
    for fitness 28–31
    for high cholesterol 28
    for weight control 254
Beta carotene
    for Alzheimer's disease 68
    for atherosclerosis 21
    for cancer 21
    for forgetfulness 21, 68
    for macular degeneration 81
    for rheumatoid arthritis 21
    See also Carotenoids *and* Vitamin A
Biceps
    exercises for 210
    illustration of 130
Bicycling
    best places for 169

bicycle types for 170
    calories burned during 230
    clothing for 171
    equipment for 171
    nature trails for 217
    water for 171
    See also Aerobics
Biotin
    for diabetes 77
    for energy 30
Bird watching 216
Blood pressure, *see* High blood pressure
Body fat, *see* Weight control
Body mass index (BMI) 234
Bone loss, *see* Osteoporosis
Brassica vegetables
    for cancer 73
    See also Broccoli
Breakfast, for weight control 247
Breast cancer 73, 117
    See also Cancer
Broccoli
    for osteoporosis 87
    See also Brassica vegetables
Brown rice, for weight control 254
Buttermilk, for gum disease 96

C

Calcium
    for high blood pressure 91
    for insomnia 99
    for muscles 25
    for osteoporosis 25, 86
    for stroke 91
    for teeth 96
Calisthenics, *see* Strength training, Stretching, *and* Warming up
Cancer 72–75
Canoeing 172, 216
    See also Aerobics
Carbohydrates
    for energy 14–15
    for insomnia 98–99
    See also Refined grains *and* Whole grains

Cardiovascular disease, *see* Atherosclerosis, High blood pressure, High cholesterol, *and* Stroke
Carotenoids
    for macular degeneration 80–81
    See also Beta carotene, Lutein, Lycopene, Vitamin A, *and* Zeaxanthin
Cataracts 31, 37, 42
Celery, for weight control 252
Cha cha, *see* Latin Dancing
Chest muscles, *see* Pectoralis major
Chinese cuisine, *see* Asian diet
Cholesterol, *see* High cholesterol
Chromium
    for diabetes 17, 76
    for hypoglycemia 76
Cigarettes, *see* Smoking
Colon cancer 15–16, 28, 73, 117, 146
    See also Cancer
Constipation, exercise for 2
Contra dancing 221–222
    classes for 222
    for flexibility 221–222
    for muscles 221
    See also Dancing
Cramps, *see* Muscle cramps
Cross training 217
    See also Aerobics *and* Strength training
Cross-country skiing 172
    See also Aerobics
Cruciferous vegetables, *see* Brassica vegetables
Cucumbers, for weight control 252
Curcumin, for rheumatoid arthritis 89–90

D

Dairy foods
    fats and 27
    for fitness 24–28
    for osteoporosis 24

See also Milk *and* Yogurt
Dancing
    calories burned during 230
    choosing styles of 220–221
    classes for 221
    for aerobic exercise 220
    for Alzheimer's disease 118
    for flexibility 220
    for forgetfulness 118
    for muscles 220
    for osteoporosis 117, 220
    See also Aerobics
DASH diet
    for high blood pressure 47–49
    salt and 48
Dehydration 12
Deltoids
    exercises for 128–129, 204–205, 208–209
    illustration of 130–131
    stretching for 142, 143–144
Diabetes 75–77
    atherosclerosis and 75
    exercise for 4
    weight control and 75
Dieting, *see* Weight control
Diets, *see* Asian diet, DASH diet, High-protein diets, Mediterranean diet, Ornish diet, *and* Step diet
Dining out, *see* Restaurants

E

Eating out, *see* Restaurants
Eggs
    fats and 52
    high cholesterol and 40, 52
EPA (Eicosapentaenoic acid), *see* Omega-3 fatty acids
Exercise
    chest pain and 126
    for Alzheimer's disease 67, 118
    for arthritis 117
    for atherosclerosis 113, 116–117
    for back pain 117

G

Gallstones 11, 244
Gardening
  allergies and 219
  for depression 219
  for flexibility 218
  for muscles 218
  for osteoporosis 117, 219
  for weight control 218
Garlic
  for atherosclerosis 79–80
  for cancer 73
Ginger
  for osteoarthritis 84
  for rheumatoid arthritis 89–90
Glucosamine, for osteoarthritis 84
Gluteus maximus, illustration of 131
Golf
  for back problems 226
  for high cholesterol 226
  for muscles 226
  for weight control 226
  inexpensive equipment for 225
Golfing
  calories burned during 230
Gout 11, 239
Grains, *see* Refined grains *and* Whole grains
Greek cuisine, *see* Mediterranean diet
Green tea
  for atherosclerosis 79
  for cancer 73
  for gum disease 97
  for high cholesterol 79
  for osteoporosis 88
  See also Tea
Gum disease 96–97
Gyms, good locations for 194–195

H

Hair care 96–97
Hamstrings
  exercises for 129, 205–208
  illustration of 131
  stretching for 139
HDL (high-density lipoprotein) cholesterol, *see* High cholesterol
Headaches, *see* Migraines
Heart attack, *see* Atherosclerosis, High blood pressure, *and* High cholesterol
Heart disease, *see* Atherosclerosis, High blood pressure, High cholesterol, *and* Stroke
High blood pressure
  anger management and 106
  diet scam dangers and 236
  fad diets and 239
  heart attack and 79
  new guidelines for 161
  stress and 107
  weight control and 233–234
  workout safety and 161
High blood sugar, *see* Diabetes
High cholesterol 77–80
  atherosclerosis and 50
  stroke and 50
High-protein diets
  atherosclerosis and 239
  cancer and 239
  diabetes and 239
  gout and 239
  high blood pressure and 239
  high cholesterol and 239
  kidney disease and 239
  osteoporosis and 239
  stroke and 239
  See also Protein *and* Weight control
Hiking 155, 216
  See also Aerobics *and* Nature walks
Horse chestnut, for varicose veins 93
Horseback riding 216
Hydrotherapy, for rheumatoid arthritis 90
Hypertension, *see* High blood pressure

I

Indian cuisine, *see* Asian diet
Insomnia 98–100
  high cholesterol and 98
  stress and 99
Insulin resistance, *see* Diabetes
Iron, for energy 33
Irritable bowel syndrome (IBS),
    stress and 106
Italian cuisine, *see* Mediterranean
    diet

J

Jenny Craig 241
  See also Weight control
Jogging, *see* Running
Jumping rope 172
  See also Aerobics

K

Kidney stones 11, 13

L

Latin dancing
  for balance 223
  for flexibility 223
  for muscles 223
  See also Dancing
Laughter, *see* Smiling
LDL (low-density lipoprotein) cho-
    lesterol, *see* High cholesterol
Leg muscles, *see* Hamstrings *and*
    Quadriceps
Legumes, *see* Beans
Lettuce, for weight control 252
Line dancing
  classes for 224–225
  for aerobic exercise 224
  for balance 224

for forgetfulness 224
  for muscles 224
  See also Dancing
Low-calorie diets 241
Low-fat diets 240–241
  See also Ornish diet *and* Weight
    control
Lutein
  for macular degeneration 81
  See also Carotenoids
Lycopene
  for asthma 70
  for cancer 73
  for macular degeneration 81
  for prostate cancer 21
  for stomach cancer 21
  See also Carotenoids

M

Macular degeneration 80–82
Magnesium
  for asthma 70–71
  for atherosclerosis 80
  for insomnia 99
  for muscle cramps 30
  for muscles 30
  for osteoporosis 88
  for stress 99
Massage, for depression 110
Meat
  atherosclerosis and 37, 40
  cancer and 40
  high cholesterol and 40
  weight control and 40
Meditation
  for anxiety 107
  for high blood pressure 107
  for high cholesterol 107
  for mental health 107
  for pain 107
  for stress 107
Mediterranean diet
  alcohol and 58
  antioxidants and 56
  fats and 57

Mediterranean diet *(continued)*
fiber and 56
for atherosclerosis 56–58
for cancer 56
for high cholesterol 56
trans fats and 57
whole grains and 56
Melatonin, for insomnia 98
Memory loss, *see* Forgetfulness
Migraines 42, 106
Milk
for high blood pressure 91
for stroke 91
See also Dairy foods
Monounsaturated fats
for arthritis 38
for atherosclerosis 38, 57
for cancer 38
for cholesterol 38
for diabetes 38
for forgetfulness 38
for high blood pressure 38
for high cholesterol 52, 57
for rheumatoid arthritis 90
for skin care 94
Morning stiffness 134
Movement therapy 173–189
See also Pilates, Tai chi, *and*
Yoga
Muscle cramps 134
Muscle loss 191

N

Nail care 96–97
National Senior Games 4, 231
Nature walks 217
See also Aerobics *and* Hiking
Negative-calorie foods
for weight control 252
See also Celery, Cucumbers, *and*
Lettuce
Niacin
for insomnia 99
See also B vitamins

Nuts
for atherosclerosis 37
for cataracts 37
for high cholesterol 37
for osteoarthritis 37
weight control and 37

O

Obesity, *see* Weight control
Obliques
exercises for 128–129, 211–212
illustration of 130
Olive oil
for atherosclerosis 57
for high cholesterol 57
for rheumatoid arthritis 90
for skin care 94
See also Monounsaturated fats
Omega-3 fatty acids
for Alzheimer's disease 68–69
for atherosclerosis 77, 89
for cancer 74
for diabetes 76
for high blood pressure 32
for high cholesterol 32, 77
for macular degeneration 81
for rheumatoid arthritis 89
for skin care 93
for stroke 91
See also Fish *and* Fish oil
Omega-6 fatty acids
Alzheimer's disease and 68
cancer and 74
macular degeneration and 81
skin care and 94
Onions
for atherosclerosis 79–80
for cancer 73
Orange juice, for weight control
252
Oranges, for weight control 254
Ornish diet
exercise and 53
fats and 54
for atherosclerosis 53–54

Ornish diet *(continued)*
  for high blood pressure 53–54
  for high cholesterol 53–54
  meat and 53
  See also Low-fat diets *and*
    Weight control
Osteoarthritis 83–84, 135
Osteoporosis 85–88, 135

P

Partially hydrogenated oil, *see*
    Trans fats
Pectoralis major
  exercises for 128, 201–202
  illustration of 130
Pets
  for fitness 217
  for stress 110
Phosphorus, for osteoporosis 26
Pilates
  classes for 188–189
  clothing for 184
  equipment for 184
  exercise examples of 185–188
  for atherosclerosis 174
  for balance 173–174, 184
  for flexibility 173–174, 184
  for muscles 173–174, 184
  for posture 184
  for strength training 174
  for stress 174
Polyunsaturated fats
  for high blood pressure 32
  for high cholesterol 32, 52
Popcorn, for weight control 254
Portion size, *see* Serving size
Potassium
  for atherosclerosis 80
  for fitness 22
  for high blood pressure 48, 61
  for muscles 22
  for osteoporosis 88
  for stroke 92
Potatoes, for weight control 254
Power walking 152–153

See also Aerobics
Prayer, for stress 107
Processed grains, *see* Refined
    grains
Prostate cancer 21
  See also Cancer
Protein
  for hair care 97
  for muscles 29
  for nail care 97
  See also High-protein diets

Q

Quadriceps
  exercises for 129, 205–208
  illustration of 130
  stretching for 140

R

Refined grains
  atherosclerosis and 15
  diabetes and 15
  high cholesterol and 15
  weight control and 15
  See also Whole grains
Religion, *see* Prayer
Restaurants, weight control and
    248–249
Rheumatoid arthritis 88–90
  atherosclerosis and 88
  stroke and 88
Riboflavin, in enriched flour 16
Rowing 172
  See also Aerobics
Rumba, *see* Latin dancing
Running 172
  calories burned during 230
  for osteoporosis 117
  for ulcers 116
  for weight control 115
  See also Aerobics

S

Saccharin
  for weight control 42
  See also Artificial sweeteners
Salt
  high blood pressure and 44, 60
  osteoporosis and 60
Sarcopenia, *see* Muscle loss
Saturated fats, *see* Fats
Selenium
  for asthma 72
  for cancer 18, 74–75
  for rheumatoid arthritis 89
  for thyroid disease 18
Serving size
  for beans 29
  for meats 41, 52
  weight control and 246, 248
Shellfish
  for vitamin B12 34
  for zinc 35
Shoulder muscles, *see* Deltoids
Skating 159, 172
  See also Aerobics
Skiing, cross-country 172
Skin cancer, *see* Skin care
Skin care 93–96
Sleep problems, *see* Insomnia
Sleep, for weight control 248
Smiling
  for mental health 102
  for pain 109
  for stress 109
Smoking
  cancer and 72
  free radicals and 2
Snowshoeing 172
  See also Aerobics
Sodium, *see* Salt
Spinning 169
  See also Bicycling
Sports
  for aerobic exercise 172
  over-50 leagues and 216
  See also Aerobics
Square dancing 221–222

classes for 222
  for flexibility 221–222
  for muscles 221
  See also Dancing
Step aerobics 159, 162–164
  See also Aerobics
Step diet
  fats and 51
  fiber and 52
  for high cholesterol 50–53
Stomach muscles, *see* Abdominals
    and Obliques
Strawberries, for anxiety 107
Strength training
  arthritis and 193
  asthma and 193
  atherosclerosis and 193
  calories burned during 230
  cancer and 193
  chest pains and 198
  clothing for 196
  exercise examples of 201–212
  food and 196–197
  for back pain 201
  for bicycling 192
  for diabetes 193–194
  for golf 192
  for higher metabolism 191–192,
    201
  for muscle loss 191–192
  for osteoporosis 117, 192
  for running 192
  for sports 192
  for tennis 192
  for weight control 115–116,
    191–193, 201
  good locations for 194–195
  high blood pressure and 193, 197
  injuries and 193
  osteoporosis and 193
  pain and 198
  proper technique for 197–199
  setting a schedule for 195
  water for 196
  women and 195
Stress
  arthritis and 106
  asthma and 106

Stress *(continued)*
  atherosclerosis and 106
  free radicals and 2
  irritable bowel syndrome and
    106
  migraines and 106
  weight control and 251–253
Stretching
  exercise examples of 139–144
  for aerobic exercise 136
  for back pain 138
  for balance 133
  for flexibility 133
  for golf 133, 226
  for injuries 134, 136
  for morning stiffness 134
  for muscle cramps 134
  for muscles 133–134
  for osteoarthritis 135
  for pain 134
  for posture 134
  for sports 133, 136
  for strength training 133, 136,
    199
  for stress 138
  for walking 133, 149–150
  for water aerobics 165
  osteoporosis and 135
  proper technique for 136–138
Stroke 90–92
  high blood pressure and 91–92
Sugar
  atherosclerosis and 62
  fats and 62
  gum disease and 62
  weight control and 62
Sunburn, *see* Skin care
Sunlight
  for depression 110
  for vitamin D 27, 84, 86, 219
Swimming
  calories burned during 230
  clothing for 168
  See also Aerobics

T

Tai chi 173
  calories burned during 230
  classes for 188–189
  clothing for 179, 183
  exercise examples of 180–182
  for arthritis 174, 178–179
  for balance 173–174, 178, 183
  for flexibility 173–174, 183
  for forgetfulness 179
  for high blood pressure 178
  for muscles 173–174, 183
  for pain 178–179
  for stress 174, 179, 183
Talk test 121, 151
Target heart rate 125–126, 150
Tea
  for atherosclerosis 79
  for osteoporosis 88
  See also Green tea
Tennis 227–230
  calories burned during 230
  for balance 228
  for flexibility 228
  for osteoporosis 228
  for stress 228
  inexpensive equipment for 225
Thai cuisine, *see* Asian diet
The Zone diet, *see* High-protein
  diets
Thiamin
  for Alzheimer's disease 67
  See also B vitamins
Thyroid disorders, weight control
  and 242
Tooth decay, *see* Gum disease
Tooth loss, *see* Gum disease
Trans fats
  atherosclerosis and 43
  cancer and 43
  high cholesterol and 43
Trapezius
  exercises for 129, 204–205
  illustration of 131
Treadmills 153–154

Triceps
exercises for 128, 210–211
illustration of 131
Triglycerides, *see* Atherosclerosis
Tryptophan, for insomnia 98–99
Turmeric, for rheumatoid arthritis
89–90
Type 1 diabetes, *see* Diabetes
Type 2 diabetes, *see* Diabetes

U

Ulcers 104, 116
Ultraviolet light, skin care and 94

V

Varicose veins 93
Vegetables
for cancer 73
for fitness 18–24
for weight control 252
Vitamin A
for Alzheimer's disease 68
for atherosclerosis 79
for skin care 94
See also Beta carotene *and*
Carotenoids
Vitamin B12
for Alzheimer's disease 67
for osteoarthritis 83
See also B vitamins
Vitamin B2, *see* Riboflavin
Vitamin B3, *see* Niacin
Vitamin B6
for Alzheimer's disease 67
for insomnia 100
See also B vitamins
Vitamin C
for Alzheimer's disease 68
for asthma 70
for atherosclerosis 75, 79
for colds 20
for diabetes 75
for high cholesterol 75, 79

for iron absorption 31
for kidney disease 75
for macular degeneration 81–82
for muscles 20
for osteoarthritis 83
for skin care 95
for stroke 75
Vitamin D
for calcium absorption 86
for muscles 27
for osteoarthritis 84
for osteoporosis 27
Vitamin E
for Alzheimer's disease 39, 68
for asthma 72
for atherosclerosis 38–39, 79
for cancer 39
for macular degeneration 82
for rheumatoid arthritis 89
for skin care 94
for stroke 39
Vitamin K, for osteoporosis 87

W

Walking
calories burned during 230
for atherosclerosis 116, 146
for colon cancer 146
for constipation 116
for diabetes 117, 146
for energy 145–146
for heart attack 4
for high blood pressure 145
for high cholesterol 145
for insomnia 145–146
for osteoporosis 117
for stress 145–146
for stroke 117
for ulcers 116
for warming up 135
for weight control 145
good technique and 152
hiking and 155
museums and 217
treadmills and 153–154

Walking *(continued)*
  See also Aerobics
Waltz, *see* Ballroom dancing
Warming up
  for gardening 219
  for strength training 198
  for stretching 135, 136–137
  for walking 149–150
Water
  for fitness 11–13
  for gallstones 11
  for gout 11
  for gum disease 11
  for heartburn and indigestion 11
  for kidney stones 11
  for osteoarthritis 11
  for rheumatoid arthritis 90
  for skin care 96
  for urinary tract infections 11
  for weight control 252
Water aerobics
  calories burned during 230
  equipment for 168
  for arthritis 166
  See also Aerobics
Weight control
  fad diets and 236–241
  for atherosclerosis 233–234
  for cancer 72, 233
  for diabetes 75, 233
  for gallbladder disease 233
  for high blood pressure 233
  for osteoarthritis 233
  for rheumatoid arthritis 89
  for sleep apnea 233
  for stroke 233
  gallstones and 244
  hormones and 242
  hypothyroidism and 242
  medication and 242
  scams and 235–236
  yo-yo dieting and 238
Weight Watchers 241
  See also Weight control
Whole grains
  for atherosclerosis 15
  for cancer 15
  for diabetes 15

for diverticulosis 15
for fitness 13–18
for stroke 92
for weight control 254
See also Refined grains
Wrinkles, *see* Skin care

Y

Yoga
  calories burned during 230
  classes for 188–189
  clothing for 175
  equipment for 175
  exercise examples of 176–178
  for arthritis 174
  for atherosclerosis 174
  for balance 173–174
  for flexibility 173–175
  for high blood pressure 175
  for high cholesterol 175
  for muscles 173–174
  for stress 174–175
Yogurt
  for gum disease 96
  See also Dairy foods

Z

Zeaxanthin
  for macular degeneration 81
  See also Carotenoids
Zinc
  for energy 35
  for gum disease 97
  for hair loss 97
  for macular degeneration 35, 82